To my husband Dave, this book is for you.

# TABLE OF CONTENTS

# food to some
# poison to others

## The Food Allergy Detection Program

# TERRY TRAUB R.D.H., B.S.
### WITH A FOREWORD BY DAVID E. ALLEN, M.D.

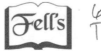

Frederick Fell Publishers, Inc
2131 Hollywood Blvd., Suite 305
Hollywood, Fl 33020
www.Fellpub.com   email: Email: fellpub@aol.com

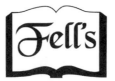

Frederick Fell Publishers, Inc
2131 Hollywood Blvd., Suite 305
Hollywood, Fl 33020
www.Fellpub.com   email: Email: fellpub@aol.com

This publication is designed to provide accurate and authoritative information in regard to the subject matter covered. This book is not intended to replace the advice and guidance of a trained physician nor is it intended to encourage self-treatment of illness or medical disease. Although the case histories presented are true, all names of patients have been changed.

Library of Congress Cataloging-in-Publication Data

Traub, Terry, 1948-
 Food to some poison to others : the food allergy detection program / by Terry Traub ; forward by David E. Allen.
     p. cm.
 Includes bibliographical references and index.
 ISBN-13: 978-0-88391-171-6 (pbk. : alk. paper)
 1. Food allergy--Diagnosis. 2. Food allergy--Diet therapy. I. Title.
 RC596.T73 2008
 616.97'5--dc22
                                    2008019485
 10 9 8 7 6 5 4 3 2 1

# FORWARD

Food allergies have gone undiagnosed for years, decades and yes, even lifetimes. The result of these undiagnosed food allergies have caused a multitude of intestinal, respiratory, skin and other problems. Discovering the offending food is not always obvious, and many labeled with asthma, "irritable bowel", eczema or other unexplained disorders never go further to look for the cause.

It is always better to find a cause for a disease. Effort is frequently required for optimal health. Exercise, proper diet, rest and stress reductions all require effort and foresight. Our different genetic makeup and exposures to various antigens in infancy make it wise to consider what food our bodies will function best with.

Food tests such as the RAST test have their place and can be helpful, but are not always reliable. For example the severe gluten allergy called celiac disease will be missed by the RAST test but would be discovered by the method in this book. There is now a specific blood test for Celiac Sprue but not for the many other food allergies.

This book has the potential for transforming a person with an unknown food allergy from disease to wellness. What is food to some is poison to another; we are not all created the same. Discovering "your" poison is worth the time and effort.

—David E. Allen, M.D. Internal Medicine.

# PREFACE

It's been many years since I wrote "The Food Allergy Detection Program." Before I decided to republish this book, I researched to see if a need still existed. Surely with all the new advances, the need was minimal. The results of my research demonstrated that there was still a very great need. New blood tests can show gluten sensitivity, but for most food allergies, the "Gold Standard" is still the elimination diet. This is when possible offending food from the individual's diet is eliminated and a food challenge follows. That is what this book's aim will be. When I first wrote this book, it was because of my sons' allergy problems and the trials I went though. I assumed other parents were having the same problems as I did. Now my husband has the problem. While my sons were somewhat compliant, my husband is not! He will not eat tofu; he is a meat and potatoes man. Therefore I have changed my approach. The diet is now for parents, busy individuals on the go, Baby Boomers, the X-generation and others who are experiencing new food allergies later in life. I have created short cuts that will make the diet easier to follow.

Food allergies are difficult to identify because of the many reactions an individual might have and the reaction time between the exposures to the allergen. A typical reaction time is one to ten hours, and with latent reactions, such as gluten (wheat) it can take up to 72 hours. So to identify the offending food, one needs first to eat foods that are considered safe. Then add possible suspect foods. During this time, a very accurate diary of the times involved between ingestion of the food and the reactions should be completed.

This book will focus on the food agents causing the allergies. It is a handbook, elimination diet and cookbook all in one. It has an easy to follow diary to help discover problem foods. The book also touches on "Irritable Bowel Syndrome" and "GERD" (gastric reflux). Some recipes and preparation for the recipes are with these individuals in mind. It is hoped that the information in this book will create an awareness of the specific cause and lend information to the parent, individual and physician in attempting to find the correct diagnosis. This book is to be used with your physician to collect information and data. By working together, the cause of the food allergies will be discovered. I have also included in this book easy cooking remedies to help the cook in the family cope with the challenge of cooking Allergy-Free.

Best of Luck
—Terry Traub, RDH, B.S.

# ACKNOWLEDGMENTS

So many people were involved with the creation of this book. Their suggestions, diligence, and culinary help brought the book to its fruition.

I would like to express my gratitude to Dr. David E. Allen, who examined my manuscript for its medical accuracy and his support in the completion of the book.

My thanks to the many recipe contributors. These include: Lillian Garvin, Nancy Deuell, my sister Veronica Holland for her help in the salad section, Donald and Norma Kessler, Denise Mc Breen, Victoria O'Conner, Doris Thurston, and David Traub.

My special thanks to Joanne Angerame. Her expertise with the dessert, breads, and cookie section was especially helpful.

I would like to thank all my tasters: Dr. Timothy O'Connor and staff, the Upper Pinebrook Potluck Group, my husband, family, and friends.

I would also like to thank K. Andrew Kent, whose efforts and guidance initiated the commencement of this book.

I would like to thank Elena Solis for all her hard work and creativity on this book.

# INTRODUCTION

The ingestion of food is normally a simple, satisfying process to most people. Food allergies occur when a person's immune system generates an anti-body response to the ingested food. These individuals, especially children, may exhibit abnormal or exaggerated reactions to food. These reactions manifest themselves in a variety of ways and can cause much discomfort. Symptoms of food allergies in children can take the form of runny noses, coughing, asthma, itchy throat, diarrhea, abdominal pain, excessive sweating, mucus in the chest, eczema, constipation, and vomiting. In adults, the symptoms of food allergies may take the form of hay fever, asthma, diarrhea, itchy eczema, headaches and migraines, dizziness, eye problems, heartburn, and gastric distress. These are all frequently confused with other diseases. Such a variety in symptoms and the time period involved for reaction to the food by the individual makes immediate diagnosis by the physician almost impossible.

Food allergies can be temporary, permanent or delayed. Temporary good allergies will disappear after a period of abstinence and slow reintroduction. A permanent allergy is a fixed allergy, which will not disappear even after years of avoidance. Masked allergy or delayed allergy is a latent reaction to a food. This reaction can take anywhere from 12 to 72 hours before symptoms appear.

Some allergies to food seem to be more prominent at certain times of the year. This seems to be due to two reasons. First, many foods are seasonal and available in higher quantities at certain times. Secondly, some allergies have properties that when combined with a certain food during a pollinating time of the year may produce a reaction, while the ingestion of the food during the nonpollinating season produces no reaction.

Because food allergies are often misdiagnosed for years, they can lead to other more serious diseases such as: Osteoporosis, irritable bowel syndrome (IBS), internal hemorrhaging caused by Crohn's disease and/or ulcerative colitis, pancreatic disease, miscarriages, internal lymphoma, and other intestinal and various malignances. Certain autoimmune disease can also be associated with some of these food allergies. They are: Insulin-dependent diabetes, lupus, thyroid disease, Addison's disease, rheumatoid arthritis and Sjogen's syndrome.

The following chart indicates common allergy manifestations:

## ALLERGY MANIFESTATIONS

| Symptoms | Diarrhea & Grastric Distress | Migraines | Headaches | Eczema |
|---|---|---|---|---|
| Possible Food Causes | Wheat and gluten foods (oats, barley, rye) Raw meat Pineapple juice Cokes/Coffee Citrus Juices Dairy Products Grain Liquors Some vegetables | Monosodium Glutamate Salts Cheses Chocolate Ham Dairy Products Nuts Pineapple Various alcoholic drinks: Beer, Wine(especially red) Grain alcohols and liquers | Same as Migraines Caffeine Sugar Wheat | Dairy Products Wheat Products Citrus Foods High Sugar Foods |

| Symptoms | Hives & Itching | Swelling | Anaphylactic Shock | Sinus & Nasal Congestion | Asthma |
|---|---|---|---|---|---|
| Possible Food Causes | Chocolate Tomatoes Strawberries Citrus Gluten Foods | Honey Egg Whites | Egg Whites Shrimp/ Crab Lobster | Dairy Products Chocolate Beer/Wine | Multiple Foods The List is Endless |

# THE MECHANICS OF FOOD ALLERGIES, INTOLERANCE, AND MALABSORPTION

The mechanics of food allergies in the body are not fully understood. The immune system of the body is a highly complex defense mechanism that helps us to fight infections and other problems. It does this by identifying any foreign object or invader and instructing the body's white cells to fight. However, in some individuals the body identifies non-toxic substances as toxic and instructs the white cells to react, thereby creating the allergic reaction to a normal food. A typical food allergy is immediate. It takes the form of asthma, hives, migraine, and anaphylactic attacks. These reactions are usually easy to figure out. It is the latent reactions that are difficult.

Food intolerance is an exaggerated but not immediate reaction to foods. The symptoms of intolerance that develop after eating a specific food are: stomach distress, diarrhea, eczema, migraines, and vomiting. Many foods such as apples, melons, cucumber, onions, cabbage, coconuts, coffee, sodas and certain spices, are known for their difficulty in digestion. If an individual is lacking the proper enzyme to protein associated with the food, then the food is not absorbed by the body and excreted in the form of diarrhea. Lactose intolerance falls in this category, as does Gluten (wheat) intolerance. The proteins involved are lactose and casein, for milk; gluten or gliadin for wheat; ovalbumin in the egg white; and zein in corn.

Malabsorption is another type of food related difficulty. It is a digestive problem associated with food. While it is not considered a food allergy it is one of the most experienced problems associated with various food allergies and other related diseases. An individual with malabsorption fails to properly absorb the necessary nutrients minerals and vitamins from the food they ingest. The body is left wanting more food because it does not utilize the food and its properties. Symptoms of diarrhea, gas, fatigue, loss of weight or the opposite, obesity, dry skin and bruising, depression, gastric reflux are just some of the symptoms associated with this syndrome. The important thing is finding the cause. Some possible causes are poor nutrition, Celiac disease, damage to the intestinal walls from high doses of antibiotics, Irritable Bowel syndrome, Crohn's disease, and other digestive disorders. This returns us to the food. Which foods started the whole disease process?

# TESTING FOR FOOD ALLERGIES AND INTOLERANCES

1. The Skin Prick Test. This test has two solutions. One control (negative control) is diluents and the other control (positive control) is a histamine solution. A drop of allergen solution is placed on the forearm. It is then introduced into the body by scratching the arm. The reaction is evaluated after 15 minutes. The test is quite reliable for house dust mites, grass pollen, and cat and dog allergens. However, the test is less reliable with food allergens. This is due to the difficulties encountered in the preparation of the numerous food extracts and the instability and standardization of the extracts once they are prepared.

2. Intracutanous Test. The intracutanous test is performed by intradermal (under the skin) injections into the skin with the suspected allergen. These tests are rarely used except for diagnosis of drug or venom allergy (i.e. bee venom).

3. Patch Test. The Patch test is widely used in the diagnosis of allergic contact dermatitis. Most of these tests are standardized and easy to administer. The allergens are placed on the skin. There is a 48 to 72 hour reaction to the allergen.

4. Serum Allergy Specific IgE Concentration Test. In this radioactive test called RAST (radioallergosorbent test), the patient's serum is tested to see if allergen specific IgE binds to immobilized allergen. This test works if the allergen is still in the individual's blood stream but can give false positives.

5. Blood Tests for Serum Specific IgE Allergens. Enzyme Linked Immunosorbent Assay (ELISA) is a non-radioactive method, which utilizes the enzyme labeling of anti-IgE, the antigen is added to the patient's serum in a fluid form.

Both the Rast and ELISA test are more accurate than those in the past and can be up to 92% accurate for inhaled allergen, less depending on what kind of food allergen.

6. Food Challenge. While there have been many advances in the research of food allergies. Food challenge is still considered the "Gold Standard" of the medical community. Ideally the food challenge should be a double blind test. This can only be done in the hospital where neither the individual nor the investigator knows what is being served. This is both time consuming and expensive.

7. Food Elimination Diet. This is a nonallergic diet that the individual may ingest without the necessity of fasting. The individual limits the number and types of food he/she may eat. This "A- Diet" is used until symptoms of distress from allergies are gone. Then suspect foods are added one at a time and a strict diary is kept of any reactions and times of the reaction.

# DISCOVERING YOUR POISONS
## OR
# HOW THIS ALLERGY
# FREE DIET WORKS

First and foremost, the need to get you or your loved one out of pain and distress becomes the goal. To do that, an ALLERGY FREE DIET needs to be implemented. The AF-FREE DIET will have foods that are not known to be allergic or prepared in such a manner that negative response is limited. This diet will not deal with any anaphylactic foods. SPECIAL NOTE: Individuals with anaphylactic problems should not try this diet. Follow only what your physician instructs.

The foods that are known to cause most of the trouble are: milk and dairy products (except for goat and sheep milk products); wheat, gluten and flours such as: barley, rye, spelt, kamut and triticate; eggs (usually the yolks); corn (especially corn starch); chocolate (usually with milk or it's fat); and pork (again it is probably the fatty cuts of pork: ham, bacon etc.).

The above foods will not be used in this diet. If they are included for any reason it will be noted. The safest food we will be using will be rice, and other hypoallergenic foods. The rice used will be from packages not from boxes that are processed. With rice and other safe foods to eat, the suspected allergy foods will then be eliminated for 12 days. What we are trying to do is give the body almost 2 weeks to heal itself before inducing any allergens. During these 12 days, the foods eaten will be divided into four-day sections. Poultry will be eaten one day; Fish on another day; the next day will be Vegetarian; and the last day will be a Meat day. The same food groups will be eaten on the same days to make diary recording easier. The poultry, meat and fish all need to be lean with no or little fat. The beef and turkey should range-free if possible and the poultry is to be organic (white meat only). If possible, the fish should be caught and not farm-raised. These foods and others will be ingested in sequence. Strict adherence to the sequence is important for elimination and identification of all offending foods.

After the twelve days, the individual will then add the first suspected food. In our first test we want to try eggs and egg yolks. Make sure your physician is aware that you are undertaking this testing. Some foods you will only need to take once, like eggs and egg yolks. Others like wheat you will need to eat for three days. Then return to the AF-Free Diet for four days. Try another possible allergy food for three days and return again to the AF-Free Diet again for four days. Make sure that you are keeping a diary of what you ate and all the symptoms and the times. Tests for allergy will be in this order: Eggs and egg yolks, corn and cornstarch, gluten and wheat products, and milk or dairy products. Dairy products in this book refer to cow's milk. Sheep and goat milk and cheese will be used instead of cow's milk. Chocolate and pork is tested minimally in this book. See sheets for diary attached. Keep in mind that testing order is important as egg yolks, egg whites, and cornstarch are in everything! Once the testing gets past these all too possible suspects, it will be easier to make and buy premade food.

One last note: There is no such thing as an Allergy-free food. Everyone is allergic to something. And as hard as this book will try, someone out there will be allergic to foods that are considered safe. Please bear this in mind when utilizing this book.

# PREPARATION FOR THE AF-FREE DIET

Due to the fact that many of the recipes for the AF-Free Diet are from health food and/or organic food stores such as Whole Foods™, new pantry items are required. While you may feel these items are expensive, they are less expensive than trips to the hospital. Also some precooking will need to be done. While gluten free breads are available in most stores, some have egg whites and others have cornstarch. Read the labels carefully!

## NECESSARY PANTRY ITEMS

**Beans**
Pinto (kidney)
Garbanzo beans (chickpeas) great for making hummus
Cannellini beans (white navy beans)
**Beef**
Kosher meats (produced without milk products)
Lean beef (for hamburger and other recipes you will need ground chuck and other lean beef)
Range feed beef (hormones in the beef can cause a multitude of problems)
**Cereals**
Puffed rice
Puffed millet
Quinoa cereals
Pure buckwheat
Also any cereal that states it is gluten and corn free
**Cheeses**
Cheeses made from goat's milk
Cheeses made from ewe's milk
(See Ingredient Glossary)
**Eggs**
Golden harvest Egg Replacer
Ener-G Egg Substitute
Other egg substitutes
Egg whites

**Fish**

Canned salmon

Canned tuna (packed in fresh water)

White fish like tilapia, basa, sole, snapper and cod.

Fresh salmon, halibut, scallop, and trout if possible

**Flours**

Amaranth flour

Arrowroot flour

Garbanzo Bean flour

Potato flour

Potato starch

Sorghum flour

Tapioca flour

White Rice Flour

Brown Rice Flour

All Purpose GF Baking Flour (Red Mill brand contains: Garbanzo bean flour, potato starch, tapioca, white sorghum flour, and fava bean flour.)

Arrowhead Mills- Beware this product contains cornstarch. You cannot use it until after you test for corn.

**Fruit**

Buy fresh or canned in its own juices. Do not buy any canned fruit in heavy or light syrup. This is corn syrup.

**Grains**

Brown rice, long grain white rice, basmati rice

Arborio Italian rice, used for Risotto

Wild rice

Rice pasta (can be found as lasagna, macaroni, penne, spiral and spaghetti)

Millet

Buckwheat (Kasha)

Oats (make sure it has not been contaminated with processing)

**Liquids**

Rice Milk

Almond Milk

Soy milk (There are various types manufactured)

Non- citrus juices (such as cranberry, check for corn syrup)

Herbal teas (no caffeine)

Non-Gluten beers (Redbridge, Bard's Tale Beer-Dragon's Gold and

New Grist Beer)
Bottled Water
Wines (those containing no sulfates)

**Mayonnaise**

Eggless Mayonnaise (Haines or Featherweight brands-contains egg yolk)
Vegenaise (contains soy)

**Meats**

Very lean ground chuck for hamburger
Very leans cut of beef
Lean lamb

**Nuts**

Almonds (from the rose family)
Pine Nuts (it is really a seed from the stone pine family)
Pistachio Nut (it is seed from the pistachio tree)

**Oils and Margarines**

Canola oils
Grape seed oil(good for searing meat and use at medium to high heat cooking)
Almond oil(same as above but high heat cooking)
Olive oil
Margarines made without corn or milk

**Poultry**

Lean and natural chickens, skinless, no dark meat
Range-grown turkeys (some dark ground meats)

**Seasonings and Spices**

Rice miso
Kosher salt
Sea Salt
Gluten free herbs and spices
Tamari for soy sauce (Eden Organic and San-j Organic, are both wheat-free)

# PRELIMINARY COOKING AND PREPARATION

By buying and cooking ahead of the AF-diet you will eliminate excessive time in the kitchen. One of the first things you will need to make is: homemade bread, gravies, lots of barbecue sauce for grilling, sauces, cookies, and toast points (also used as croutons). Rice and millet breads are available in the stores. There are two types: frozen and fresh sealed. Both are AF-diet safe. Though some sealed breads have cornstarch in them. Ener-g™ rice bread loafs are now corn-free. The frozen breads are very hard breads and need to be toasted to eat. I found that brushing rice bread with various oils and baking them in the oven makes the bread tasty. Homemade bread and some bread made at health food stores also may contain allergic elements. So until egg and corn is ruled out, this bread cannot be included in the AF-diet. Rice, pastas, risotto, potatoes and potato dishes are the main starches that the diet will work with. Some items that should be prepared or bought before beginning the diet are:

1. Rice Breads (Ener-g has a great commercial rice bread that is not frozen)
2. Rice crackers and thins for breading, brown rice tortillas
3. Salad dressings ( Italian, Roquefort, or French)
4. Homemade maple syrup* or store bought without corn starch. Most health food stores now contain "Pure Maple syrup". Rice syrup is now available in stores and can be used instead of corn syrup.
5. Veggie mayonnaise (Vegenaise is a good example)
6. Flours other than wheat. Most health food stores carry these flours. Flours are listed in "Necessary Pantry Items Section".

# FOODS NOT ALLOWED ON THIS AF-DIET

1. Breads or baked items containing following items: wheat, rye, barley, bulgur, wheat-based semolina, spelt, kamut, wheat starch, triticale, gluten or durum flour.
2. Corn, corn starch, corn syrup
3. Eggs, egg yolks, egg by products (egg whites will be used as an egg substitute)
4. Citrus fruits
5. Chocolate, coffee, anything with caffeine in it, teas unless it is decaffiened
6. Alcohol beverages: hard liqueur, wine (boutique wines without sulfates are okay), beer (three beers Redridge, Dragon's Gold, and New Grist are okay) and ales
7. Cow's milk, any by product of milk: curds, whey, casein, rennet, ghee, lactose, lactulose, whey and casein hydrolysates, lactalbumin, (sheep and goat's milk allowed)
8. Nuts: especially walnuts and pecans (almonds, pine nuts, and pistachios are okay)
9. Chewing gum, some candies (please read labels)
10. Fatty meats: ham, bacon, prosciutto, fatty cuts of beef
11. Margarine and butter containing corn products or cow's milk
12. Crustaceans of any form: lobster, crab and shrimp
13. Monosodium glutamate seasoning

# QUESTIONS AND ANSWERS

1. Do I need to strictly stay on the diet? Yes, straying off the diet will produce different results, thereby invalidating the information gathered during the diet.

2. Can I eat at restaurants? That is a tricky question. A good number of restaurants are offering Gluten free meals, but they still may have eggs, corn, and dairy products in the meal. My advice is if you know the restaurant owner or chef, maybe, but on the whole I would advise against it. There are now restaurants chains that offer gluten-free menus. This doesn't help with the rest of the allergies, but it is a start. Some restaurants request you order a week in advance so they can accommodate you. Refer to section "On the Road" page # 39.

3. Will I spend much time in the kitchen? This is something that I am hoping to eliminate. There are some great health food stores throughout the United States. "Whole Foods" is one of the largest. 25 years ago, being able to buy and find allergy free foods prepared was impossible, but now it is easier. However, there will be some things you need to prepare prior to starting the AF-diet. See the Preliminary Cooking section.

4. Where do I find the ingredients and foods necessary for the diet? Before just health food stores carried the items need for the AF-diet. Now some supermarkets and smaller markets are ordering specialty items. Ask your grocer if you cannot find the item you need or go to a health food store in your area.

5. Do I have to prepare the food in any special way? Most of the recipes are very specific on how to prepare the food. For example, most turkey and chicken recipes are skinless and use dark meat sparingly. Note: you may cook the poultry in its skin to retain the moistness, but remove before eating.

6. Should I take vitamins supplements during the AF-diet? Ask your doctor for advice on vitamins. If he does consider them necessary, be careful of the vitamins you buy. Some manufacturers use cornstarch as a binder, others use wheat. Read the label!

7. Can I substitute shortening or butter for margarine in any of the recipes? First, let's get our terms straight. Shortening is a universal term for solidified vegetable oils, lard, salt pork, beef or lamb. The flavor variety obtained from the various forms of shortening is due to the fatty acids. Saturated fatty acids that are usually solid at room temperature come from animal sources. Unsaturated fatty acids, in-

cluding polyunsaturated, are generally liquid at room temperature. These are cold pressed vegetable oils, such as olive oil. Hydrogenated vegetable shortening is an unsaturated vegetable oil that has had hydrogen added to it to change it from liquid to solid. Doing so changes the oil from unsaturated to saturate.

Now to answer the question, no you may not use shortening in place of margarine if it is saturated, whether animal or vegetable. People with gluten problems and individuals with "Irritable Bowel Syndrome" cannot absorb solid fats. Shortening will cause stomach distress to these and other allergy individuals. But, there are nonhydrogenated, Trans fat-free shortenings available at health food stores, Spectrum and Smart Balances are two manufacturers of this type of shortening.

# ❧ THE AF-DIET ❧

## THE 12 DAY AF WORKSHEETS

### DAY 1 POULTRY DAY

| Menu | Food Family and Substitute | Time Ingested | Reactions | Time of Reactions |
|---|---|---|---|---|
| **Breakfast** | | | | |
| Rice/ | | | | |
| Buckwheat Pancakes* | Grass family | | | |
| Maple syrup* | Maple family (Pure maple syrup from health stores okay) | | | |
| Fresh apricots | Plum family (do not use any fruit in syrup) | | | |
| **Lunch** | | | | |
| Barbecue Chicken* | | | | |
| Rice chips (available at health food stores) | | | | |
| Fresh nectarines | | | | |
| Dessert (optional) | | | | |
| **Dinner** | | | | |
| Turkey/ Chicken Gravy* | | | | |
| Sliced Roasted Turkey (can be bought from store) | | | | |
| Turkey Stuffing* | | | | |
| Asian Cranberry topping*(or organic cranberry sauce) | | | | |
| **Dessert (optional)** | | | | |

*Note: All dishes marked with asterisks
(\*) have recipes in the book and can be located by consulting the index.*

### DAY 2  FISH DAY

| Menu | Food Family and Substitute | Time Ingested | Reactions | Time of Reactions |
|---|---|---|---|---|
| **Breakfast** | | | | |
| Riceola* | Grass family-millet | | | |
| Banana | Banana Family | | | |
| Cranberry juice | Blueberry family | | | |
| **Lunch** | | | | |
| Tuna Sandwich | Fish Family | | | |
| Pears, sliced | | | | |
| Potato chips, baked | | | | |
| **Dinner** | | | | |
| Tarragon | | | | |
| Oven-baked Fish* | Fish family- snapper, cod, tilapia | | | |
| Green salad* | Composite family | | | |
| Roquefort dressing * | Meat family (sheep milk) | | | |
| Skillet potatoes* | Nightshade family | | | |
| Dessert (optional) | | | | |

### DAY 3 VEGETARIAN DAY

| Menu | Food Family and Substitute | Time Ingested | Reactions | Time of Reactions |
|---|---|---|---|---|
| **Breakfast** | | | | |
| Apricot Nut Bread* | Plum family | | | |
| Cantaloupe | Gourd Family | | | |
| Beverage | | | | |
| **Lunch** | | | | |
| Portabella mushroom sandwich* | Mushroom family | | | |
| Green salad | Composite family | | | |
| **Dinner** | | | | |
| Vegetable Sheppard Pie* | | | | |
| Spicy Spinach salad* | Goosefoot & composite families | | | |
| Dessert (optional) | | | | |
| Beverage | | | | |

**DAY 4 MEAT DAY**

| Menu | Food Family and Substitute | Time Ingested | Reactions | Time of Reactions |
|---|---|---|---|---|
| **Breakfast** | | | | |
| Cooked millet | Grass family | | | |
| Maple Syrup*(or commercial-pure) | | | | |
| Blueberries | Blueberry family | | | |
| **Lunch** | | | | |
| Sliced beef | Meat family | | | |
| Feta Beet salad* | Goosefoot family | | | |
| Toasted rice bread | | | | |
| **Dinner** | | | | |
| Salisbury Steak | Meat family | | | |
| Green salad | | | | |
| Dessert (optional) | | | | |

**DAY 5 POULTRY DAY**

| Menu | Food Family and Substitute | Time Ingested | Reactions | Time of Reactions |
|---|---|---|---|---|
| **Breakfast** | | | | |
| Oatmeal | Grass family | | | |
| Peaches, sliced | Plum family | | | |
| **Lunch** | | | | |
| Turkey burgers* | Fowl and grass family | | | |
| Carrot Cake* | Parsley family | | | |
| **Dinner** | | | | |
| Hot Turkey Sandwiches* | | | | |
| Turkey/Chicken gravy)* | | | | |
| Brussels sprout | Mustard family | | | |

## DAY 6 FISH DAY

| Menu | Food Family and Substitute | Time Ingested | Reactions | Time of Reactions |
|---|---|---|---|---|
| **Breakfast** | | | | |
| Rice/ | | | | |
| Buckwheat pancakes | Grass family (Rice cereal okay) | | | |
| Maple syrup* | Maple family (commercial "pure maple" okay) | | | |
| Sliced apples | Rose family | | | |
| **Lunch** | | | | |
| Tuna Melt | Fish family | | | |
| Potato salad* | Nightshade family | | | |
| Sliced carrots | | | | |
| **Dinner** | | | | |
| Company | | | | |
| Halibut* | Fish Family | | | |
| Risotto | Grass family | | | |
| Green salad* | Composite family | | | |
| Dessert | | | | |

## DAY 7 VEGETARIAN DAY

| Menu | Food Family and Substitute | Time Ingested | Reactions | Time of Reactions |
|---|---|---|---|---|
| **Breakfast** | | | | |
| Cooked Buckwheat | Buckwheat family | | | |
| Maple Syrup* (commercial "pure maple" okay) | | | | |
| Apricots | Rose family | | | |
| **Lunch** | | | | |
| Avocado Provencal* | Laurel family & | | | |
| Salad* | Composite family | | | |
| Sliced Cucumbers | Gourd family | | | |
| Dessert (optional) | | | | |
| **Dinner** | | | | |
| Salad | Composite family | | | |
| Stir-Fried Vegetables | | | | |
| Sautéed Zucchini* | Gourd family | | | |
| Dessert (optional) | | | | |

## DAY 8  MEAT DAY

| Menu | Food Family and Substitute | Time Ingested | Reactions | Time of Reactions |
|------|------|------|------|------|
| **Breakfast** | | | | |
| Cooked millet | Grass family (rice cereal) | | | |
| Cranberry sauce* | | | | |
| Beverage | | | | |
| **Lunch** | | | | |
| Spicy Spinach salad* | Goosefoot & composite families | | | |
| Commercial rice bread | Grass family | | | |
| Dessert (optional) | | | | |
| **Dinner** | | | | |
| Easy Hamburger & Rice* | Meat & Grass families | | | |
| Skillet beets | Goosefoot family | | | |
| Dessert (optional) | | | | |

## DAY 9 POULTRY DAY

| Menu | Food Family and Substitute | Time Ingested | Reactions | Time of Reactions |
|------|------|------|------|------|
| **Breakfast** | | | | |
| Riceola* | Grass family | | | |
| Peaches | Rose family | | | |
| Beverage | | | | |
| **Lunch** | | | | |
| Turkey, sliced | Fowl Family | | | |
| Green salad* | Composite family | | | |
| French dressing* | | | | |
| Dessert (optional) | | | | |
| **Dinner** | | | | |
| Turkey/sausage Loaf* | | | | |
| Romano Carrots | | | | |
| & Cauliflower* | Mustard family | | | |
| Rice Dish* | Grass family | | | |
| Dessert (optional) | | | | |

**DAY 10 FISH DAY**

| Menu | Food Family and Substitute | Time Ingested | Reactions | Time of Reactions |
|---|---|---|---|---|
| **Breakfast** | | | | |
| Rice pudding* | Grass family | | | |
| Plums | Plum family | | | |
| **Lunch** | | | | |
| Pasta salad* | | | | |
| Rice chips | | | | |
| Hummus | | | | |
| **Dinner** | | | | |
| Barbecue Salmon | Fish family | | | |
| Green salad* | Composite family | | | |
| French dressing* | | | | |
| Dessert (optional) | | | | |

**DAY 11 VEGETARIAN DAY**

| Menu | Food Family and Substitute | Time Ingested | Reactions | Time of Reactions |
|---|---|---|---|---|
| **Breakfast** | | | | |
| Rice or | | | | |
| Buckwheat pancakes | Grass family | | | |
| Maple Syrup* | Maple family (commercial "pure maple" syrup okay) | | | |
| Honeydew melon | Gourd family | | | |
| **Lunch** | | | | |
| Cream of Tomato Soup* | | | | |
| Potato Picnic Salad* | Nightshade family | | | |
| Sliced Apples | Apple family | | | |
| **Dinner** | | | | |
| Zucchini Boats* | Gourd family | | | |
| Rice Pilaf* | Grass family, Rose family | | | |
| Carrot-Raisin Salad* | Parley & grape family | | | |
| Dessert (optional) | | | | |

30

**DAY 12 MEAT DAY**

| Menu | Food Family and Substitute | Time Ingested | Reactions | Time of Reactions |
|---|---|---|---|---|
| **Breakfast** | | | | |
| Rice pancakes | Grass family | | | |
| Maple Syrup* | | | | |
| Blueberries | | | | |
| **Lunch** | | | | |
| Sliced roast beef | | | | |
| Feta Beet Salad* | Goosefoot & meat family | | | |
| Banana | Banana family | | | |
| Dessert (optional) | | | | |
| **Dinner** | | | | |
| Beef burgundy* | Meat family | | | |
| Rice pasta | Grass family | | | |
| Garlic green beans | Bean family | | | |
| Dessert (optional) | | | | |

31

# TESTING FOR EGGS, CORN, WHEAT, AND MILK

To test for a food allergy once the individual is healthy without symptoms, then it is time to test. We will start with eggs, then corn, wheat, milk, chocolate, and pork. The first four are most important. Once eggs and corn is tested then more foods are open to the individual. This is because gluten free baking goods are usually made with egg whites, egg yolks, and cornstarch. Once the egg and corn testing is done, then products containing eggs and cornstarch can be added to the AF-diet. You will find more products you can buy instead of making them.

### TESTING FOR EGGS

For three days, add eggs: For example add Eggs (fried, scrambled, etc) for breakfast. Add eggs, instead of egg substitute to recipes. Use eggs for egg salad, omelets and as a binder in meatloaf. Return to the AF-diet for four days. If you find yourself reacting to eggs find out if it is the yolk or the white. Most egg substitutes still have egg whites. Most commercial breads have egg whites in them.

### TESTING FOR CORN

For three days, add corn products: for example add corn syrup to maple syrup for breakfast; add fresh or creamed corn for lunch and choose Deep Fried Fish* for dinner. Return to the AF-Diet for four days. If you find yourself reacting to corn or cornstarch well I'm sorry. Cornstarch is in EVERYTHING. You have the most difficult food allergy to deal with. One company, Ener-g has many corn-free products. You will find them at www.ener-g.com. Contact a physician or allergy specialist to assist you in your diet.

### TESTING FOR WHEAT

For three days, add wheat products: for example, use regular flour bread for breakfast and lunch sandwiches, and choose Turkey Divan* for dinner. Return to AF-Diet for four days. This allergy or intolerance will not show its effects until the third day and will continue with the distress for three days! If you find you are reacting to wheat or gluten, you may have celiac disease. Check with your doctor. Celiac Disease organization is the biggest and most active associations in the nation. Go into any health food store or large health food stores like "Whole Foods" and you will find a plethora of products waiting for you. There are so many new products and foods being produced that the minute this book is published its list of gluten products will be out of date.

## TESTING FOR MILK PRODUCTS

For three days, add dairy products: for example eat cottage cheese for breakfast, pizza for lunch, and Turkey Goulash for dinner. Usually hard cheeses are easier to digest than soft cheeses, ice cream and heavy creams. The reaction might be immediate so be prepared. Return to AF-Diet for four days. If you find you are reacting to cow milk products then you have the easiest problem to control. There are so many non-dairy products around that it will not be hard for you to adapt. My youngest son will simply ask for no sour cream in most of his meals at restaurants and asks if the cheese is cooked. Normally cooked cheese will not cause a problem, but find out what you need to do that works. Using dairy digestive products will not work if you over use them. Only use them on special occasions or when you are at friends and do not know what is in the meal. Goat and sheep cheeses are getting very popular and can be found everywhere. My favorite is Gouda goat cheese. You will find them in my mushrooms in the appetizer section.

## TESTING FOR CITRUS, CHOCOLATE, PORK AND ANY OTHER SUSPECTED ALLERGEN

Follow the same procedures as Egg, Corn, Wheat and Milk (Dairy Products).

# TESTING WORKSHEETS

## TESTING FOR EGGS WORKSHEET

| Menu | Food Family and Substitute | Time Ingested | Reactions | Time of Reactions |
|------|---------------------------|---------------|-----------|-------------------|
| **Breakfast** | | | | |
| **Lunch** | | | | |
| **Dinner** | | | | |

## TESTING FOR CORN WORKSHEET

| Menu | Food Family and Substitute | Time Ingested | Reactions | Time of Reactions |
|------|---------------------------|---------------|-----------|-------------------|
| **Breakfast** | | | | |
| **Lunch** | | | | |
| **Dinner** | | | | |

## TESTING FOR WHEAT WORKSHEET

| Menu | Food Family and Substitute | Time Ingested | Reactions | Time of Reactions |
|------|----------------------------|---------------|-----------|-------------------|
| **Breakfast** | | | | |
| **Lunch** | | | | |
| **Dinner** | | | | |

## TESTING FOR MILK WORKSHEET

| Menu | Food Family and Substitute | Time Ingested | Reactions | Time of Reactions |
|------|----------------------------|---------------|-----------|-------------------|
| **Breakfast** | | | | |
| **Lunch** | | | | |
| **Dinner** | | | | |

# SOURCES OF EGGS, CORN, WHEAT AND MILK

Years ago with the first book manufactures were not required to disclose everything that was in the product. Happily that has changed and many items are now easier to read. The best new law starting in 2008 is the requirement of stating if the product is "Gluten Free". This will make easier to find food that are A-Diet safe. There is time needed for reading labels, but it will not be so complicated. The following lists include examples of foods containing possible allergens unless otherwise stated. These are not complete lists for the manufacturing techniques are forever changing.

## SOURCES OF EGGS

Malted chocolate drinks
Frostings and icings
Hollandaise sauce
Custards
Some salad dressing
Soufflés
Marshmallows
Meringues
Cream pies
Sausages
Eggnog

Pastas, noodles
Jelly roll, donuts, glazed rolls
Some pancakes and waffle mixes
French toast
Hamburger mix
Mayonnaise
Bavarians and mousses
Tartar sauce
Sherbets
Breads
Ice cream

## SOURCES OF CORN

Beer, ale
Gin, whiskey
Carbonated drinks
Instant teas
Crackers
Sherbets
Jam, jellies
Corn tortillas
Doughnuts
Commercial pie crusts
Some non-dairy whipped toppings
Hominy
Frostings
Peanut butter
Monosodium glutamate

Catsup
Some baking powders
Fruit canned in syrup
Instant coffees
Ice cream
Corn cereals
Custards, puddings, Jell-O
Commercial cakes and cookies
Syrups
Some non-dairy creamers
Corn chips
Popcorn
Chili
Cornstarch
Caramel coloring

Note: Cornstarch is used as a base in many brands of aspirin, vitamins, toothpastes, and glue. A corn base is found in most paper products such as wax paper and paper cartons.

## SOURCES OF WHEAT

Beer, ale
Gin, whiskey
Malted beverages
Doughnuts
Rolls
Cookies
Biscuits
Puddings
Sausages
Commercial special breads
Matzo
Rye
Some yeasts
Farina, graham
Wheat starch

Flours: all-purpose, spelt, white,
Flours: wheat,
Bran products
Wheat germ
Pumpernickel
Chocolate candy bars
Pretzels
Some commercial gravy mixes
Commercial cornbread
Gluten flour and breads
Bologna
Bisquick and pancake mixes
Some ice creams
Noodles, pasta
Vermicelli

As of 2008 all United States manufacturers are suppose to label whether there are wheat ingredients in their products.

## SOURCES OF MILK

Milk – whole, low-fat, fat-free
Milk – condensed
Milk – powdered and evaporated
Buttermilk
Creams – sour and heavy
Ice cream
Ice milk
Milk chocolate
Cheeses (except those made from Ewe's,
Goat's, or Buffalo's milk)
Creamed foods
Scrambled Eggs
Butter
Some margarines

Pie crusts
Cookies
Bisquick and pancake mixes
Crackers
Biscuits
Doughnuts
Bavarians and mousses
Soufflés
Au gratin food
Soup and soup bisque
Bologna
Sausage
Nougat
Fritters

The lists above are an incomplete list. Labels need to be read to ensure that the allergen foods are included in the ingredients.

# BEFORE YOU START THE AF-DIET

In this time in our society, I have found some habits that are distressing. We have forgotten how to eat! Most individuals seem to have gastric reflux (which is not being tested for in this book). So I am including some do's and don'ts to protect you from eating improperly. It takes our digestive systems about 15 hours to digest the food we eat. If we go to bed too soon after our final meal for the day, the food will not get improperly digested and food following gravity will end up back in your mouth instead of in the intestine where it belongs. Give the stomach the time it needs to digest. The second problem is people do not chew their food long enough. This is what happens. There is a little flap in our esophagus (called the lower esophageal sphincter) that allows the food to go on to the stomach. It opens every 25 to 27 seconds. If someone is stuffing food down their mouth without chewing or only chewing for 5 seconds, all the food gets trapped on top of this flap and will weaken the flap so much that food that already went through the flap will go backwards up into your mouth with acid from the stomach. Another problem is taking pills or vitamins at night, if you take these pills just before you go to bed without waiting at least an hour or two the pill will lie in the esophagus over night causing holes in the esophagus. Drinking lots of water after taking a pill should be on the container instructions. Being a Dental Hygienist by profession, during the last ten years I have noticed more and more people with decay in the back edges of their molars. The acid coming up from the stomach will cause decay on the second molars or teeth closest to the throat. People will wash their mouths out after an attack of gastric reflux, but will forget to brush. Tooth decay can develop within three months after gastric reflux attacks begin, not to mention holes in the esophagus.

**THE DO'S**

Do chew you food more (about 25 times)
Do wait 3 hours after eating before bed
Do buy fresh vegetables
Do read all labels
Do buy new flours
Do see your physician if you suspect GERD

**THE DON'Ts**

Do not eat late at night
Do not drink large amounts
between bites
Do not buy processed foods
Do not drink caffeine or cokes
Do not eat at fast foods
restaurants
See you Dentist if you
have GERD

# ON THE ROAD

When traveling with an allergic individual or if it is just you, it is a frustrating experience to try and find anything to eat on the road. The following chapter will give you some tips and information to make your choices easier.

In these busy times, we are constantly on the road, whether it is for business, family get- to-gathers, or sport events. As parents, many of us are constantly driving our children to their sport events or other activities. These events take time getting there and time getting back. All of us at some point, need to eat. The problem is finding a restaurant that is safe and will not cause allergic distress. You can carry safe foods with you, but at some point a restaurant will be needed.

## THE GOOD NEWS

Because of the strength and activities of gluten-free organizations, many restaurants are aware of allergy-free menus and have stepped up to fill a need. By just going on the Internet and looking for gluten-free restaurants you will find many offerings. The following are just a sample of the plethora of information available:

**CHAIN RESTAURANTS OFFERING GLUTEN-FREE (ALLERGY-FREE) MEALS:**

**Alabama:** Carrabbas Italian Grill, Bonefish Grill, Chili's, On the Border, Out-Back Steakhouse, P.F. Chang's China Bistro, Ted's Montana Grill.

**Alaska:** Chili's, Outback Steakhouse, Romano's Macaroni Grill.

**Arizona:** Carrabbas Italian Grill, Chili's, First Watch, On the Border, Outback Steakhouse, Pasta Pomadoro, P.F. Chang's China Bistro, Peiwei Asian Diner, Romano's Macaroni Grill, Uno Chicago Grill, Z'Tejas Southwestern Grill.

**Arkansas:** Carrabbas Italian Grill Chili's, Claim Jumper, On the Border, Peiwei Asian diner, Romano's Macaroni Grill.

**California:** Chili's, Claim Jumper, On the Border, Outback Steakhouse, Pasta Pomadoro, P. F. Chang's China Bistro, Peiwei Asian Diner, Romano's Macaroni Grill, Uno Chicago Grill, Z'Tejas Southwestern Grill.

**Colorado:** Carrabbas Italian Grill, Bonefish Grill, Chili's, Claim Jumper, On the

Border, Outback Steakhouse, P.F. Chang's China Bistro, Romano Macaroni Grill, Ted's Montana Grill.

**Connecticut:** Carrabbas Italian Grill, 99 Restaurant, Bugaboo Creek Steakhouse, Chili's, Fresh City, On the Border, Outback Steakhouse, P.F. Chang's China Bistro, Romano's Macaroni Grill, Ted's Montana Grill, Uno Chicago Grill.

**Delaware:** Bugaboo Creek Steakhouse, Chili's, Outback Steakhouse, P.F. Chang's China Bistro, Romano's Macaroni Grill.

**District of Columbia:** Austin Grill, Chili's, Legal Seafood, Outback Steakhouse, P.F. Chang's China Bistro, Romano's Macaroni Grill.

**Florida:** Carrabbas Italian Grill, Bonefish Grill, Chili's, First Watch, Legal Seafood, On the Border, Outback Steakhouse, P.F. Chang's China Bistro, Peiwei Asian Diner, Romano's Macaroni Grill, Uno Chicago Grill.

**Georgia:** Carrabbas Italian Grill, Bonefish Grill, Bugaboo Creek Steakhouse, Chili's, On the Border, Outback Steakhouse, P.F. Chang's China Bistro, Romano's Macaroni Grill, Ted's Montana Grill, Wildfire Restaurants.

**Hawaii:** Chili's, Outback Steakhouse, P.F. Chang's China Bistro, Romano's Macaroni Grill.

**Idaho:** Carrabbas Italian Grill, Chili's, On the Border, Outback Steakhouse, P.F. Chang's China Bistro, Romano's Macaroni Grill.

**Illinois:** Carrabbas Italian Grill, Bonefish Grill, Chili's, Claim Jumper, On the Border, Outback Steakhouse, P.F. Chang's China Bistro, Romano's Macaroni Grill, Ted's Montana Grill, Uno Chicago Grill, Wildfire Restaurants.

**Indiana:** Carrabbas Italian Grill, Biaggi's Ristorante Italiano, Bonefish Grill, Chili's, On the Border, Outback Steakhouse, P.F. Chang's China Bistro, Romano's Macaroni Grill, Ted's Montana Grill, Uno Chicago Grill.

**Iowa:** Biaggi's Ristorante Italiano, Bonefish Grill, Chili's, On the Border, P.F. Chang's China Bistro, Romano's Macaroni Grill.

**Kansas:** Carrabbas Italian Grill, Bonefish Grill, Chili's, First Watch, On the Border, Outback Steakhouse, P.F. Chang's China Bistro, Peiwei Asian Diner, Romano's Macaroni Grill, Ted's Montana Grill.

**Kentucky:** Carrabbas Italian Grill, Biaggi's Ristorante Italiano, Chili's, First Watch, On the Border, Outback Steakhouse, P.F. Chang's China Bistro, Romano's Macaroni Grill.

**Louisiana:** Carrabbas Italian Grill, Bonefish Grill, Chili's, On the Border, P.F. Chang's China Bistro, Uno Chicago Grill.

**Maine:** 99 restaurants, Bugaboo Creek Steakhouse, Chili's, On the Border, Outback Steakhouse, Uno Chicago Grill.

**Maryland:** Carrabbas Italian Grill, Austin Grill, Biaggi's Ristorante Italiano, Chili's, First Watch, Legal Seafood, Outback Steakhouse, P.F. Chang's China Bistro, Peiwei Asian Diner, Romano's Macaroni Grill.

**Massachusetts:** Carrabbas Italian Grill, 99 Restaurants, Bugaboo Creek Steakhouse, Chili's, Fresh City, Legal Seafood, On the Border, P.F. Chang's China Bistro, Romano's Macaroni Grill, Uno Chicago Grill.

**Michigan:** Carrabbas Italian Grill, Bonefish Grill, Chili's, On the Border, Outback Steakhouse, P.F. Chang's China Bistro, Romano's Macaroni Grill, Uno Chicago Grill.

**Minnesota:** Biaggi's Ristorante Italiano, Chili's, P.F. Chang's China Bistro, Peiwei Asian Diner, Romano's Macaroni Grill, Wildfire Restaurants.

**Mississippi:** Bonefish Grill, Chili's, On the Border, Outback Steakhouse, Romano's Macaroni Grill.

**Missouri:** Carrabbas Italian Grill, Chili's, On the Border, Outback Steakhouse, P.F. Chang's China Bistro, Peiwei Asian Diner, Romano's Macaroni Grill, Ted's Montana Grill, Uno Chicago Grill.

**Montana:** Chili's, Outback Steakhouse.

**Nebraska:** Carrabbas Italian Grill, Biaggi's Ristorante Italiano, Bonefish Grill, Chili's, Outback Steakhouse, P.F. Chang's China Bistro, Romano's Macaroni Grill, Ted's Montana Grill.

**Nevada:** Carrabbas Italian Grill, Bonefish Grill, Chili's, Claim Jumper, On the Border, Outback Steakhouse, P.F Chang's China Bistro, Peiwei Asian Diner, Romano's Macaroni Grill, Z'Tejas southwestern Grill.

**New Hampshire:** Carrabbas Italian Grill, 99 Restaurants, Bugaboo Creek Steakhouse, Chili's, Fresh City, Outback Steakhouse.

41

**New Jersey:** Carrabbas Italian Grill, 99 Restaurants, Charlie Brown Steakhouse, Chili's, Fresh City, Legal Seafood, On the Border, Outback Steakhouse, P.F. Chang's China Bistro, Romano's Macaroni Grill.

**New Mexico:** Carrabbas Italian Grill, Chili's, Outback Steakhouse, P.F. Chang's China Bistro, Peiwei Asian Diner, Romano's Macaroni Grill, Uno Chicago Grill.

**New York:** 99 Restaurants, Bugaboo Creek Steakhouse, Charlie Brown Steakhouse, Chili's, On the Border, Outback Steakhouse, P.F. Chang's China Bistro, Romano's Macaroni Grill, Ted's Montana Grill, Uno Chicago Grill.

**North Carolina:** Carrabbas Italian Grill, Biaggi's Ristorante Italiano, Bonefish Grill, Chili's, On the Border, Outback Steakhouse, P.F. Chang's China Bistro, Peiwei Asian Diner, Romano's Macaroni Grill, Ted's Montana Grill, Uno Chicago Grill.

**North Dakota:** Chili's, Outback Steakhouse.

**Ohio:** Carrabbas Italian Grill, Bonefish Grill, Chili's, First Watch, On the Border, Outback Steakhouse, P.F. Chang's China Bistro, Peiwei Asian Diner, Romano's Macaroni Grill, Uno Chicago Grill.

**Oklahoma:** Carrabbas Italian Grill, Bonefish Grill, Chili's, First Watch, On the Border, Outback Steakhouse, P.F. Chang's China Bistro, Peiwei Asian Diner, Romano's Macaroni Grill.

**Oregon:** Chili's, Claim Jumper, Outback Steakhouse, P.F. Chang's China Bistro, Romano's Macaroni Grill.

**Pennsylvania:** Carrabbas Italian Grill, 99 Restaurants, Bugaboo Creek Steakhouse, Chili's, First Watch, Legal Seafood, On the Border, Outback Steakhouse, P.F. Chang's China Bistro, Romano's Macaroni Grill, Ted's Montana Grill, Uno Chicago Grill.

**Rhode Island:** Carrabbas Italian Grill, 99 Restaurants, Bugaboo Creek steakhouse, Chili's, Fresh City, Legal Seafood, On the Border, Outback Steakhouse, P.F. Chang's China Bistro, Romano's Macaroni Grill, Ted's Montana Grill, Uno Chicago Grill.

**South Carolina:** Carrabbas Italian Grill, Bonefish Grill, Chili's, Outback Steak house, P.F. Chang's China Bistro, Romano's Macaroni Grill, Uno Chicago Grill.

**South Dakota:** Chili's, Outback Steakhouse.

**Tennessee:** Carrabbas Italian Grill, Bonefish Grill, Chili's, On the Border, Outback Steakhouse, P.F. Chang's China Bistro, Peiwei Asian Diner, Romano's Macaroni Grill.

**Texas:** Carrabbas Italian Grill, Chili's, On the Border, Outback Steakhouse, P.F. Chang's China Bistro, Peiwei Asian Diner, Romano's Macaroni Grill, Uno Chicago Grill, Z'Tejas Southwestern Grill.

**Utah:** Carrabbas Italian Grill, Biaggi's Ristorante Italiano, Chili's, Outback Steakhouse, P.F. Chang's China Bistro, Peiwei Asian Diner, Romano's Macaroni Grill, Z'Tejas Southwestern Grill.

**Vermont:** Chili's, Outback Steakhouse, P.F. Chang's China Bistro.

**Virginia:** Carrabbas Italian Grill, Austin Grill, Bonefish Grill, Chili's, First Watch, Legal Seafood, On the Border, Outback Steakhouse, P.F. Chang's China Bistro, Romano's Macaroni Grill, Ted's Montana Grill, Uno Chicago Grill.

**Washington:** Bonefish Grill, Chili's, Claim Jumper, Outback Steakhouse, P.F. Chang's China Bistro, Romano's Macaroni Grill, Z'Tejas Southwestern Grill.

**West Virginia:** First Watch, Chili's, Outback Steakhouse, Uno Chicago Grill.

**Wisconsin:** Carrabbas Italian Grill, Biaggi's Ristorante Italiano, Bonefish Grill, Chili's, Outback Steakhouse, P.F. Chang's China Bistro, Romano's Macaroni Grill, Uno Chicago Grill.

**Wyoming:** Chili's, Outback Steakhouse.

# THE BAD NEWS

Fast food restaurants are what every child wants to eat. Unfortunately, they are unhealthy, fattening and for the allergic individuals-toxic. I have put together information that I hope will be helpful to those individuals who find their only choice might be a fast food restaurant.

## THE BETTER CHOICES

### Chipotle
This fast food restaurant has the motto "Our Food with Integrity". It is the ONLY restaurant that serves beef, chicken, and pork without hormones or antibiotics. Most of their meat is naturally raised. Their beans are organically grown. Their sour cream (dairy product) does not contain the hormone rBGH. The food is often served with burritos either corn or flour (both considered allergens until tested). So while this restaurant sound like an excellent fast food restaurant, it does not work until testing is done.

### In and Out Burger
This fast food restaurant is better than most. It has complete control of the beef from the time the cow is slaughtered till it arrives at each restaurant. There are no additives or fillers in the beef. Their lettuce, onion, and potatoes are all fresh. The fries are not coated before they are fried. Unfortunately, like all fast foods we are dealing with Trans fatty acids in the frying oil. The bun of the hamburger contains wheat and gluten. In and Out have in their normal menu the "Protein Style Burger". This features the burger wrapped in lettuce. Their condiments do have some additives. The pickle relish and ketchup both contain corn syrup. The mayonnaise of course contains eggs. The milkshake are gluten-free, but do contain dairy products and corn syrup. The lemonade is gluten-free, but contains corn syrup. The ice tea is Allergy-free.

### Baja Fresh
This fast food restaurant advertises that their food is fresh without fillers. However, when asked they responded that they actually use corn syrup often in their prod-

uct. Food items containing corn syrup are: the Breaded fish, Charbroiled Chicken, Chicken taquitas, Corn tortillas, Chips and strips, Enchilada salsa, Fish salsa, flour tortillas (contain gluten), Grilled peppers and onions, Ranch Dressing (also contains dairy products), Rice Salsa Rojas, and Steak taquitos. They put milk products in their breaded fish and flour tortillas.

### El Pollo Loco
This fast food restaurant advertise a "healthy dining" menu. Some are special requests such as the Flamed –Grilled Chicken Breast and The Boneless skinless Chicken Breast meal. These meals contain the chicken breast with fresh steamed vegetable, garden salad and house salsa. The salad dressing and tortillas can be omitted. Also, some al la carte sides are safe. The pinto beans have no fillers, the fiesta cheese (contains dairy) contains no gluten. The Spanish rice, which one would think is safe, is flavored with soy sauce containing wheat.

## THE OKAY CHOICES

### Wendy's
Wendy's advertises their product to be "waaaay better than Fast Food". They are however, restrictive in allowing their information to be published. Therefore, I can only refer to their website (www.wendyscom) for specific information. There you will find an ingredient list that is updated periodically. In their information, they state that some of their hamburgers and chicken recipes are gluten-free, but are surrounded by wheat buns and other ingredients. They have a wide assortment of a la carte items, some seem to be gluten-free but again with added products like eggs and cheese this is not Allergy Free. Their condiments are like all the other Fast Food Restaurants noted. They contain corn products and eggs.

### Arby's
This fast food restaurant has a few choices. The roast beef can be eaten without the bun. The Home fries (small, medium or large), marinara sauce, and potato cakes are all without allergens. Their ketchup has corn syrup in it and the honey- mustard sauce contains egg. All their chicken is coated with egg and wheat (gluten).

45

## POOR CHOICES

### McDonald's

While the Quarter Pounder beef patties may be 100% beef and safe, everything around the patties is NOT. The Big Mac sauce contains wheat, eggs and soy. The bun is of course wheat. The ketchup and pickle relish contains corn syrup. The mayonnaise contains eggs. The rest of the menu has the same problems. The Chicken patty contains wheat and egg, the Crispy Chicken Breast contains wheat, even the Grilled Chicken Breast fillet contains wheat. The fries are coated with wheat and milk. The only safe item in this restaurant is the side salad with Newman's Own Low Fat Balsamic Vinaigrette.

### Taco Bell

Taco Bell has more ingredients in every item on their menu that any of the other restaurants. Their seasoned beef contains cornstarch, soy and gluten. The Carne Asada Steak and Spicy Chicken and other entrees, contains corn by- products. Their chili and fire sauce contains gluten. The Pepper Jack sauce contains milk and egg products. The pizza sauce contains corn syrup. All the fries are coated with wheat.

### Jack In the Box

Like McDonald's and Taco Bell, the food items at this fast food restaurant, contains a multitude of ingredients. The Beef Regular Taco and the Beef Monster Taco contain corn syrup, wheat and soy. It is cooked in frying shortening. The Chicken Breast Strip, Crispy Chicken Strips, Chicken Fajita Patty, and Spicy Chicken Breast all contain cornstarch or corn flour, milk, wheat (gluten) and soy. The Chicken Roast Fillet contains cornstarch, milk products, soy and Maltodextrin. The Country Crock Spread (also found in supermarkets) contains whey and milk products, wheat (gluten), and soy. The hash browns contain corn flour. The Curly fries and Potato Wedges contain wheat (gluten), corn flour and cornstarch. The Sausage Patty contains Monosodium Glutamate. The Sirloin Beef Patty contains milk and soy. The Stuffed Jalapenos contain wheat (gluten), corn flour, whey and milk products. I really couldn't find a safe food item at this restaurant.

**Panda Express**
I wish this restaurant was safe but it isn't. Panda Express states the NONE of its dishes are gluten-free and will not give out its ingredients.

Burger King, Dell Taco, Carl's Jr. and Sonic Drive-in all have some or all of the above mentioned problems.

# THE PICNIC BASKET

Both my boys were good in sports, so as a result we on the road a great deal. We either were going to local baseball games or regional baseball and tennis matches. When we had to stay overnight at any location, I would bring the picnic basket and a cooler. Inside would be different goat and sheep cheeses, allergy-free crackers, potato salad, cole slaw, vegetables, fruit, gluten-free cookies and other items for the boys to try that they hadn't ever tried before. We would then go to a beach, lake or park for our picnic after the sports event. I asked each boy, who are now grown, what special item do they remember about the picnic basket. The answer from my youngest was the most interesting. He says he always thinks of herring in wine sauce when he thinks of picnics. That was a little different from the potato salad answer I imagined.

# AF-DIET COOKBOOK

## INTRODUCTION

When first faced with the fact that convenience foods, basic grains, breads and dairy products cannot be used in menu planning, any cook would be dismayed. But with a little practice, patience and planning, all problems can be overcome.

The object of this recipe section is to guide the cook into a new era of discovery. Not all allergy cookery is bland and unattractive; in fact just the opposite. Meals can be delicious and safe. To achieve this end, I will be making specific notes in the recipes. I have focused the recipes to include "Irritable Bowel Syndrome" problems, especially the need for soluble fibers. Soluble fibers include: oatmeal, pasta, rice, potatoes, soy, nuts, beans, lentils, and bananas to name a few. Insoluble fibers include: raw fruits and vegetables, raw greens, raw sprouts and seeds, fruit and vegetables with tough skins like green peppers, peas, celery, onions, broccoli, cabbage and more. You will find that I will either cut these ingredients finely or I will precook the insoluble fiber so that it is digestible. I am also suggesting that when eating a meal, "EAT THE SOLUBLE FIBER FIRST!! In other words, eat some of the potatoes or rice first then the meat. This is so the soluble fiber will stabilize the colon and intestine for the other foods to follow. In salads I will suggest adding soluble fiber like garbanzo beans or croutons (made from rice flour). I am also suggesting that the individual eats the salad last or after eating some rice or potatoes.

This recipe section includes recipes that were invented and gathered from our grandparents, friends and recipes from other countries with few allergy problems. I hope you find this book an adventure in cooking.

## LEGEND

The recipes in this cookbook section are coded in three different ways:
Those recipes that are considered safe to eat during the Allergy-Free Diet and afterwards for maintenance will be marked with:

• AF (Dairy-free [means the recipe does not contain milk products from cows; it will however has milk products from goat or sheep], Egg-free, Corn-free, Gluten-free [Wheat-free])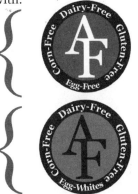

• AF (Dairy-free, Egg-free**[means there are egg whites in the recipe], Corn-free, Gluten-free [Wheat-free])

• Those recipes to be used during the testing period will marked with the letter T, for example: T (Testing for Eggs—Dairy-free, Corn-free, Gluten-free)
• Those recipes that simply state what they do not contain. They will list the eliminated ingredients under the title, such as Dairy-free, Egg-free, or Corn-free, or Gluten-free [Wheat-free])

All dishes marked with (*) are located in the recipe section and can be found by consulting the recipe index.

## TERRY'S FLOUR BLEND

Most of the cakes and tea breads in this book will be made with a special combination of flours. I have the flours individual or as a group in the flour blend. It will save time if you pre-blend the flours and have the mixture stored in an airtight container for future use.

To make 5 cups of the flour blend, mix the following flours:
2 cups white rice flour
1 ½ cups brown rice flour
1  cup sorghum flour
1/3 cup + 2 teaspoons potato starch
1/3 cup + 2 teaspoons tapioca flour

I will usually use 1 3/4 cup in most of the recipes and remove ¼ cup to save. That is because in some recipes you will need the ¼ cup flour and in others you will not.

# 🍳 APPETIZERS & DIPS 🍳

## HUMMUS

Most Hummus bought at grocery stores, I found had too much lemon juice in it. The homemade version is always the best and you can add your favorite seasonings to it.

### AF (Dairy-free, Egg-free, Gluten-free, Corn-free)

1 (15 ounce) can garbanzo beans
2/3 cup tahini sauce*
2 tablespoons olive oil
1/3 cup white wine
1 to 2 garlic cloves, minced
1/8 crushed red pepper

Process all ingredients in food processor until smooth. Add a little water if it gets too thick. Chill before serving. Hummus goes well with raw vegetables.

**Serves 8**

*Tahini Sauce is found in most Middle Eastern markets or the international section of grocery store. If you use the version in this book in the DRESSINGS AND SAUCES section omit the garlic.

### Variations:
1. Roast Red Pepper Hummus: add 3 Tablespoons roasted red pepper to mixture, reduce the wine added.
2. Add artichoke hearts to Hummus.

## DAVE'S PEPPER HUMMUS

**AF (Dairy-free, Egg-free, Corn-free, Gluten-free)**

½ can (15 ounce) garbanzo beans, drained
3-4 red roasted peppers (15 oz jar)
2 to 3 peperoncini rings
2 teaspoons lemon
2 garlic cloves, minced
1/8 teaspoon cumin
½ teaspoon salt
2 tablespoons water
2 to 3 tablespoons tahini
2 tablespoons olive oil
   dash to 1/8 teaspoon cayenne pepper
   dash crushed red pepper

Add all ingredients in food processor. Process until smooth, about 40 seconds. Chill for 4 hours or overnight. Serve with vegetables.
**Serves 4**

## QUICK SPICY CHIPOTLE BEAN DIP

This is an easy dip to do and tasty. My husband loves this with corn or rice chips

**AF (Dairy-free, Egg-free, Gluten-free)**

1/3 of (15 ounce) can of garbanzo beans
½ of (15 ounce) can of black beans
1 to 2 chipotle peppers in adobo sauce, plus at least 2 tablespoons sauce
2 tablespoons olive oil
2 tablespoons water (if needed)

Using vinyl gloves, cut chipotle peppers in half to remove seeds. (If you want the bean dip very hot omit this part.) Mix ingredients together in food processor for 30 to 40 seconds. Heat dip in microwave for 30 seconds covered with plastic wrap. Serve with chips.
**Serves 4-6**

## GUACAMOLE DIP

Avocados are a very good source of soluble fiber. This is good for individuals with "IBS". To help the problem further, I am precooking the onions and chilies.

**AF (Dairy-free, Egg-free, Corn-free, Gluten-free)**

3 to 4 ripe avocados, skin removed and seed removed
½ cup onion, finely chopped and microwave 30 seconds
1 teaspoon, minced garlic
½ teaspoon salt
½ cup stewed tomatoes
1 teaspoon wine vinegar
3 tablespoons tomato paste
1 small can (4 ounces) green chilies, chopped, microwave for 30 seconds

In medium size bowl, mash the avocados in to a paste. Add all other ingredients. Mix well. Chill before serving. Serve with Rice chips.
**Serves 8**

## CAPONATA

This mixture is excellent on toast points. Recipe for toast points to follow.

**AF (Dairy-free, Egg-free, Corn-free, Gluten-free)**

2 medium eggplants, unpeeled, cut into 1-inch cubes
¾ cup olive oil
2 large onions, chopped
½ cup green pepper, chopped
1 cup celery, chopped
1 cup chopped fresh tomatoes
2 tablespoons capers
1/3 cup red wine vinegar
2 tablespoons brown sugar
¼ cup fresh basil, chopped, or 1 teaspoon basil, dried
2 tablespoons pine nuts
¼ cup parsley,
chopped Pepper

In a large skillet, brown eggplant in olive oil. Remove and set aside. Add onions, celery, zucchini, and green pepper. Sauté' vegetables until tender. Add tomatoes and cook until tender. Add eggplant, capers, vinegar, sugar, basil, and nuts. Bring mixture to boil, reduce heat, cover and simmer for 10 minutes. Chill for 2 to 4 hours. Serve on toast points. Garnish with parsley and pepper
**Serves 8**

**TOAST POINTS**

This bread can be used for various other toppings. See note below for suggestions.

**AF (Dairy-free, Egg-free**, Corn-free, Gluten-free)**

10 slices gluten-free bread, crust removed ( special note: I found that the bread made at home, like Whole Foods 365 Everyday Sandwich mix, or Bread mix from others such as Red Mill make the best toast points. Premade gluten-free breads are too dry, except for Ener-g rice bread. This bread is not frozen and contains no corn or egg yolks. I consider this bread a Find!)
2 cups olive oil

Trim crust from bread slices. Cut bread diagonally across to make 4 pieces. Brush each side lightly with olive oil. Place in preheated 400 degree oven. Bake 3-6 minutes on one side, depending on the thickness of the bread. Remove from oven, turn pieces over. Bake for another 4 minutes or until lightly brown. Cool and store in plastic bag. Toast points can be made 2 to 3 days ahead.

**SMOKED SALMON APPETIZERS**

This is another recipe that uses toast points.

**Contains Corn (Dairy-free, Egg-free, Gluten-free)**

2 (3 ounce packages) of smoked salmon
½ container of non-dairy cream cheese (i.e. Toffutti)
4 tablespoons Italian dressing*
2 tablespoon red onion, finely chopped
½ jar capers, minced

Cut salmon into ¾ inch to 1 inch pieces. Place salmon in to small bowl and marinate in 2 tablespoons Italian dressing for 2 to 3 hours. Mix in small bowl non-dairy cream cheese and red onions*, with remaining Italian dressing. Chill for 2 to 3 hours. Place capers in food processor and process 30 seconds. Set aside. Assemble appetizer by first placing cream cheese mixture on toast points. Next place marinated salmon on top. Finally dollop mashed capers on top of salmon. Make approximately
**30 appetizers.**
*Italian Dressing can be found in Dressing and Sauces section.
*For those with IBS precooking the red onions in the microwave for 30 seconds is recommended.

## BELGIUM ENDIVE WITH ROQUEFORT CHEESE AND ALMONDS

This is one of the recipes I tested on my neighborhood potluck group. They loved this one and the following mushroom appetizer.

**(Dairy-free, Egg-free, Gluten-free)**

3/4 ounce Roquefort Sheep cheese (I especially like Socie'te' brand)
2 tablespoons non-hydrogenated margarine, room temperature
3 ounces soy cream cheese, room temperature (contains corn starch)
2 tablespoons sour cream substitute (can contain milk)
2 tablespoons organic plain yogurt (optional)
2 tablespoons roasted almonds, chopped
2 bunches Belgium Endive

Carefully pull leaves off the endive and wash them. Allow to dry on paper towels. Mix ingredients with mixer until butter smooth. Refrigerate for at least 4 hours. Spoon small amounts of Roquefort mixture on to the end of each leaf. Top with finely chopped almonds.
**Makes 30 appetizers.**

## TURKEY SAUSAGE STUFFED MUSHROOMS

My friends loved these mushrooms with the Gouda goat cheese. They had no idea they were allergy-free, and I did not give out the recipe yet.

### AF (Dairy-free, Egg-free, Corn-free, Gluten-free)

24 crimini mushrooms, stems removed and washed
2 tablespoons olive oil
2 turkey sausage, mild Italian (organic is best) skin removed, and meat broken up
¼ cup ground rice thins
3 tablespoons green onions, chopped
1 garlic clove, crushed
2 tablespoons parsley, chopped
2/3 cup goat Gouda cheese, shredded (no substitutes)

Preheat oven to 425 degrees. Place mushrooms in greased 9 by 13 baking dish. In medium skillet, heat and brown sausage. Remove from skillet and set aside. Place oil into skillet and heat. Sauté' onions and garlic in skillet for about 2 minutes. Remove from heat. Add mixture into mixing bowl; add ground rice thins, parsley, and 1/3 cup Gouda cheese. Mix together. Stuff mushrooms with mixture, top mushrooms with remaining 1/3 cup cheese. Bake covered for 8 to 10 minutes at 425. Remove top, and turn off oven, leave mushrooms in oven for 5 minutes or until cheese melts.
**Makes 24 appetizers.**

**GREEK FRIED CHEESE**

**AF (Dairy-free, Egg-free, Corn-free, Gluten-free)**

½ pound Kasseri or Kafalotysi cheese (imported from Greece)
u.s. version is made with cow's milk
flour for dusting (sorghum or rice flour)
juice of one lemon
1 tablespoon oregano
    canola oil

Cut cheese into ½ inch cubes. Dust with flour and fry in hot skillet with canola oil for 30seconds on each side. Remove from skillet. Sprinkle with lemon juice and oregano. Serve hot on beds of lettuce and sliced tomato.
**Serves 4**

**AVOCADO COCKTAIL DELIGHT**
    This is a great start to a summer meal. However, for IBS individuals, this is the last item of the meal they should eat. Also I suggest precooking the shallots in the microwave for 30 seconds.

**AF (Diary-free, Egg-free, Corn-free, Gluten-free)**

3 tomatoes, peeled and diced (use fresh only not canned)
2 small, ripe avocados
½ teaspoon sweet basil
2 tablespoons parsley, chopped
2 tablespoons shallots, minced
2 tablespoons lemon juice
2 tablespoons olive oil
    salt and pepper to taste

Peel and dice tomatoes. Discard seeds. Dice avocados. Gently combine basil, parsley, and pine nuts with tomatoes and avocado. In separate small mixing bowl, mix together shallots, lemon juice, olive oil, salt, and pepper, and pour over combined vegetables. Serve immediately in chilled cocktail glasses.
**Serves 6**

## PORCINI MADEIRA TOPPING

This is wonderful over polenta chips, recipe following.

### AF (Dairy-free, Egg-free, Corn-free, Gluten-free)

2 tablespoons canola oil
1 cup onion, chopped
½ ounce dried porcini mushrooms (found in package spice section of grocery)
¼ cup Madeira
½ cup beef broth, heated
2 garlic cloves, minced
½ teaspoon thyme
¼ teaspoon marjoram
½ teaspoon salt
¼ teaspoon pepper
 1 bay leaf

In small bowl, mix Madeira and hot beef broth. Rinse mushrooms. Pat dry. Place in bowl with broth and Madeira. Allow it to stand for 1 to 2 hours. Remove mushrooms. Drain liquid through sieve. Reserve liquid. Chop mushrooms. Add oil to sauce pan. Heat to medium heat, add onions sauté' until transparent, about 3 to 5 minutes. Add mushrooms and garlic and cook 1 minute. Add reserve liquid, spices and bay leaf. Bring liquid to boil, then turn down, cover and simmer for 10 minutes. REMOVE BAY LEAF. Using slotted spoon place mixture on cooked polenta chips. This mixture can be made 3 days ahead and reheated.
**Serves 6 to 8**

## POLENTA CHIPS

### Contains Corn (Dairy-free, Egg-free, Gluten-free)

2 refrigerated rolls of polenta, sliced into ¼ inch or less
Pam or any other vegetable spray

Preheat oven to 500 degrees. Line 2 baking sheets with foil and spray with vegetable spray. On paper towels place sliced polenta. Top with paper towel; press lightly to get liquid out of polenta. The drier the polenta, the better the chips. Place dried polenta on baking sheets. Bake polenta one tray at a time for 15 minutes. Turn polenta over. Bake another 10 to 15 minutes. Repeat with second tray. (If you have auto bake, you can bake both at the same time) Place polenta chips on warming plate. Top with Porcini Madeira mixture. Serve warm.
**Serves 8**

> Note: The Porcini Madeira mushroom mixture with the thin polenta can be a little messy. It makes a better entre for a Vegetarian Dinner. You will find it in the Vegetarian Section.

## TURKEY WRAPPED SCALLOPS

The mild taste of the scallops is a perfect foil to the salty turkey bacon.

### AF (Dairy-free, Egg-free, Corn-free, Gluten-free)

¼ cup olive oil
8 large sea scallops, cut into 4- 1 inch chunks each
8 turkey bacon slices
¼ cup Sorghum flour

Place flour in shallow bowl. Roll cubed scallops in flour and place to the side on wax paper. On cutting board, slice each bacon strip, first in half horizontally, then vertically. Each bacon strip will make 4 thin slices. Wrap turkey slice around each scallop. Secure with toothpick. Heat 12-inch skillet with olive oil to medium –high heat; place turkey wrapped scallops into skillet. Cook turning the scallops and for 20 minutes or until all areas of the scallops are lightly brown and the bacon is cooked. Serve warm.
**Makes 32 appetizers**

## ROCKAFELLER OYSTER STUFFING

Individuals who love Oysters will love this dip

### AF (Dairy-free, Egg-free, Corn-free, Gluten-free)

3 strips turkey bacon
20 to 24 spinach leaves, stems removed and cleaned
1 can smoked oysters, well drained
2 tablespoons worcestershire sauce
4 ounces soy substitute sour cream
4 ounces soy substitute cream cheese
2 tablespoons green onions, sliced
1 teaspoon lemon juice

In food processor, mince oysters and green onions. In 12-inch skillet, cook bacon until done. Remove bacon from pan. Crumble bacon.* Add 1 tablespoon oil to skillet. Then add spinach. Cook until just limp. Remove spinach from pan. Blot dry on paper towel. Mince spinach on cutting board and add spinach and ½ of crumbled bacon to oyster mixture. In separate mixing bowl beat cream cheese, sour cream, Worcestershire sauce, and lemon juice. Fold oyster mixture into cream cheese mixture. Chill for 3 to 4 hours. Use to stuff celery or as a dip. Top with remaining crumbled bacon.

*crumbled bacon- you really cannot crumble turkey bacon. I found that it is necessary to slice the cooked bacon and then mince with large butcher knife.

## WILD MUSHROOM BRUSCHETTE

### AF (Dairy-free, Egg-free**, Corn-free, Gluten-free)

$\frac{1}{2}$ loaf rice bread (Ener-g rice bread is the best, not frozen)
$\frac{1}{2}$ cup olive oil
$\frac{1}{2}$ to 1 cup shredded Manchego cheese ( sheep)
Combination of wild mushrooms, chopped (shiitake, chanterelles, oysters, portabella)
2 garlic cloves, minced
$\frac{1}{4}$ teaspoon pepper
$\frac{1}{4}$ teaspoon sage
2 to 3 teaspoon dried or 2 to 3 tablespoons of chopped thyme, or rosemary, or basil
  Dash of Port

Brush bread with olive oil. Cut each bread slice into 4 triangles. Place on cookie sheet. Sprinkle cheeses and herbs on top of bread. Place bread under broiler and cook for 2 to 3 minutes. Meanwhile, sauté mushrooms in skillet with olive oil, sage, garlic and pepper. At last minute add Port. Remove bread slices and top with mushroom mixture. Serve warm.

**Makes 24 appetizers**

### Other toppings for Bruschetta
1. Commercial salsa
2. Tomato sauce with herbs and Romano cheese (sheep)
3. Sliced figs with prosciutto (testing for pork)

## PEPPER JACK MEXICAN PIZZA

I made these for Super Bowl Sunday and they were a hit!

### AF (Dairy-free, Egg-free, Corn-free, Gluten-free)

6 Wheat-free/Gluten-free tortillas (Food for Life makes a Brown Rice version)
¾ cup of fresh tomato salsa
¾ cup of sour cream substitute
1 cup cooked chicken, chopped
½ to ¾ cup of all natural guacamole
¼ cup bell red pepper, finely chopped
1 cup goat jalapeno jack cheese
1 cup of combination of goat jack and cheddar cheeses

Preheat oven 350 degrees. Place 2 tortillas on baking sheets. Mix tomato salsa and sour cream together in small bowl. Place ¼ of salsa mixture on each tortilla. Top with ½ of chicken and combine cheeses and ½ of red peppers on each tortilla. Place next tortillas on top. Spread Guacamole on each tortilla. Place last two tortillas on top. Place last of salsa mixture on each tortilla; top with last of cheese and red peppers. Bake in oven for 15 minutes or until cheeses are melted. Cut into wedges, serve warm.

**Makes 16 appetizers**

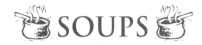 SOUPS

## BEEF STOCK

**AF (Dairy-free, Egg-free, Corn-free, Gluten-free)**

6 beef bones
½ pound inexpensive lean beef chuck
2 tablespoons oil
¼ cup onion, chopped
¼ cup celery, chopped
¼ cup carrot, chopped
3 quarts water
2 teaspoons salt
½ teaspoon pepper
1 tablespoon parsley, chopped
  Bouquet Garni*

Cut beef chuck into 1-inch cubes. In large Dutch oven, heat oil, brown beef cubes and bones. Remove from pan. Place onions, celery, and carrots into pan. Cook until tender and onions are transparent. Return beef to pan, add water, salt, pepper, and Bouquet Garni. Bring mixture to boil. Reduce heat and simmer for 3 hours. Strain through sieve. Can be stored for 2 weeks in the refrigerator.
**Makes approximately 4 cups**

## CHICKEN STOCK

### AF (Dairy-free, Egg-free, Corn-free, Gluten-free)

1 pound chicken wings
1 pound chicken necks
¼ cup oil
2 to 4 shallots, chopped
1 large leek, chopped
¼ cup celery, chopped
¼ cup carrot, chopped
1 teaspoon salt
½ teaspoon pepper
3 quarts water
  bouquet Garni*

In large Dutch oven, brown chicken wings and necks in batches. Remove chicken, add more oil if needed. Add shallots, leek, celery, carrot and sauté until tender. Return chicken to pan and add water, salt, pepper and Bouquet Garni. Bring to boil. Reduce heat and simmer for 3 hours. Strain through sieve.
**Makes about 4 cups**

## FRENCH ONION SOUP

### AF (Dairy-free, Egg-free**, Corn-free, Gluten-free)

4 onions, sliced into 1/8 inch pieces
3 tablespoons margarine, milk-free, corn-free)
1 quart beef broth
6 toast points*, cut into 4 pieces each (cubes)
½ cup grated Romano cheese, sheep, imported

In large saucepan melt margarine. Add onions and sauté until tender. Add Beef stock or broth. Bring to boil, reduce heat and simmer for 10 minutes. Pour hot soup into bowls, place toast point cubes into soup. Top with Romano cheese. Serve hot.
**Serves 6**

## BROWN CABBAGE SOUP

### AF (Dairy-free, Egg-free, Corn-free, Gluten-free)

½ cup (1 cube) margarine, milk-free, corn-free
1 ½ pounds cabbage, shredded
1 garlic clove, minced
1 tablespoon sugar
4 cups Beef Stock* or beef broth
1 teaspoon salt
¼ teaspoon pepper
¼ teaspoon allspice, ground
1 bunch parsley, chopped

In large saucepan, melt margarine. Add cabbage and garlic to pan. Sauté cabbage, turning frequently for 5 minutes. Sprinkle sugar over cabbage and simmer for 30 minutes or until the cabbage is brown all over. Add beef stock (or broth), salt, pepper, and allspice. Cover. Simmer for 1 hour or until cabbage is tender. Sprinkle with parsley. Serve hot.
**Serves 8**

## VEGETABLE BEEF SOUP

### AF (Dairy-free, Egg-free, Corn-free, Gluten-free)

1 pound beef shank
¼ cup chopped onion
2 bay leaves
2 quarts water
1 cup beef broth
1 tablespoon water
½ cup celery, chopped
½ cup carrots, chopped
¼ cup green pepper, chopped
½ cup potatoes, peeled and chopped
1 cup frozen lima bean, thawed
3 portabella mushrooms, coarsely chopped
5 peppercorns
3 tablespoons parsley, chopped

Combine beef shank, onion, bay leaves, salt, peppercorns, beef broth and water to large saucepan. Bring to boil and reduce heat. Simmer for 3 hours or until meat is tender. Remove bones and peppercorns, and skim off fat. Add remaining vegetables to broth. Cook 1 hour longer, serve hot.

**Serves 6**

## MINESTRONE SOUP

### AF (Dairy-free, Egg-free, Corn-free, Gluten-free)

2 tablespoons grape seed oil
1 pound stewing beef, cut into 1-inch cubes
½ cup sorghum flour
1 tablespoon olive oil
1 onion, chopped
4 cups beef broth
1 cup chicken broth
½ cup hot water mixed with 1 teaspoon beef bouillon
1 (15 ounce) can diced tomatoes plus juices
2 tablespoons parsley, chopped
1 teaspoon thyme
½ teaspoon salt
¼ teaspoon pepper
1 (15 ounce) can cannellini beans, drained
1 zucchini, sliced
1 cup uncooked rice pasta, spirals or elbow
½ cup Romano cheese, grated, sheep, imported

In large skillet, heat olive oil. Add chopped onions and sauté until transparent. Remove from heat. On platter mix sorghum flour with dash of salt and pepper. Dredge cubed stewing beef in flour. In 5 quart Dutch oven (or other large saucepan), heat grape seed oil. Add beef cubes and brown. Reduce heat. Add cooked onions, tomatoes and liquid, broths, water, parsley, thyme, salt, and pepper. Cook uncovered over low heat for about 1 ½ hours. Remove top, add cannellini beans, zucchini, and pasta. Cook until pasta is tender, about 30-45 minutes. Place minestrone into soup bowls, top with 1 tablespoon of Romano cheese.
**Serves 8**

## VICHYSSOISE

### AF (Dairy-free, Egg-free, Corn-free, Gluten-free)

4 large leeks, sliced
1 medium onion, sliced
2 tablespoons margarine, milk-free, corn-free
$\frac{1}{2}$ cup chicken stock* or chicken broth
3 cups boiling water
1 $\frac{1}{4}$ cups potatoes, thinly sliced
1 cup milk substitute
$\frac{1}{4}$ cup shallots, sliced

snipped chives
salt and pepper to taste

Wash leeks, cutting off their green tops, and thinly slice white parts. Melt margarine in a large saucepan, then add leeks and onions. Cover and cook over low heat for 10 minutes, but do not brown. Combine chicken broth and boiling water. Add leeks and onion, along with potatoes. Bring mixture to boil, reduce heat and simmer until potatoes are tender. Cool. Puree mixture in food processor. Add salt, pepper, and milk substitute. Chill for 3 hours. Garnish with chives.
**Serves 8**

## SPLIT PEA SOUP

### T (Testing for pork—Dairy-free, Egg-free, Corn-free, Gluten-free)

Water for soaking split peas
1 pound (2 cups dried) split peas
2 quarts water
Ham shank, skin removed
$\frac{1}{2}$ cup onion, chopped
1 cup celery, chopped
1 sprig parsley, chopped
2 teaspoons salt
$\frac{1}{2}$ teaspoon pepper
1 bay leaf

Place dried split peas in large Dutch oven. Cover with water until 1 inch above level of peas. Bring to boil and boil for 2 minutes. Remove from heat and let soak 1 to 2 hours. Drain water and add 2 quarts water and remaining ingredients. Simmer for 4 hours. Remove bay leaf and serve hot.
**Serves 6**

## CREAM OF TOMATO SOUP

### AF (Dairy-free, Egg-free, Corn-free, Gluten-free)

2 cup milk substitute (soy milk works the best)
1 (15 ounce) can tomatoes, diced
2 tablespoon margarine, milk-free, corn-free
1 tablespoon white rice flour
½ cup onion, chopped
1 teaspoon salt
½ teaspoon pepper
1 tablespoon arrowroot mixed with ¼ cup water

In large saucepan, melt margarine. Add onions and sauté until transparent. Add tomatoes and cook for 1 minute. Add flour and mix with vegetables. Slowly add milk substitute, salt and pepper. Simmer for 10 minutes. If soup needs to be thickened, add arrowroot and water combination.
**Serves 4**

## COLD TOMATO AVOCADO SOUP

### AF (Dairy-free, Egg-free, Corn-free, Gluten-free)

3 cups Cream of Tomato Soup*
1 ripe avocado, peeled and diced
1 garlic clove, minced
¼ teaspoon salt
1/8 teaspoon cayenne
1/8teaspoon pepper
¼ cup non-dairy whipped creamer
¼ cup sesame seeds
2 tablespoons parsley, chopped

In food processor puree avocado. Add avocado to tomato soup, garlic, salt, pepper, and cayenne pepper. Put soup in to bowls and allow to chill. Top soup with dollop of whipped creamer; then add sesame seeds and parsley.

## CREAMY ASPARAGUS SOUP

### AF (Dairy-free, Egg-free, Corn-free, Gluten-free)

2 tablespoons margarine, milk-free, corn-free
2 tablespoons white rice flour
1 cup chicken broth, heated
½ cup dry white wine (for **GERD** suffers, omits the wine and
    add ½ cup more chicken broth instead)
1 cup milk substitute
½ teaspoon salt
¼ teaspoon pepper
    dash white pepper
½ teaspoon dried rosemary or 2 tablespoon fresh,
chopped finely and mashed with pestle and mortar
1 pound fresh asparagus or 8 ounce package frozen,
cooked and pureed (fresh tastes better) see note*

In saucepan, melt margarine. Add flour and make roux. Stir for one minute. Slowly, add heated chicken broth to roux. Add milk substitute, wine, rosemary, salt and peppers. Add pureed asparagus. Simmer soup for 30 minutes. Add more chicken broth if soup is too thick.
**Serves 4**

Note: When using fresh asparagus, place in skillet with liquid and poach until tender. Then place in food processor to puree. This may take a little longer than the frozen version, but is worth it in taste.

## HEARTY TURKEY CHILI SOUP

### AF (Dairy-free, Egg-free, Corn-free, Gluten-free) GERD ALERT*

¾ pound turkey, ground
2 tablespoons canola oil
½ cup onion, chopped
¼ cup celery, chopped
1 carrot, peeled and grated
2 tablespoons rice flour
1 (15 ounces) can red kidney beans, drained, rinsed
1 (16 ounces) container fresh tomato salsa
1 (15 ounces) can tomato puree
1 cup beef broth
3 cups water
½ teaspoon salt
¼ teaspoon pepper
½ teaspoon chili powder
½ teaspoon ground cumin

In medium skillet, brown turkey and set aside. In large saucepan, add oil and heat. Add onions, celery, carrots and sauté until tender. Add flour and mix with vegetables. Slowly add beef broth so no lumps in broth are produced. Add water, cooked turkey, tomato puree, kidney beans, salsa, spices, salt, and pepper. Bring soup to boil, reduce heat and simmer 45 minutes.

**Serves 6**

GERD ALERT: This recipe contains tomato acid and citrus acid

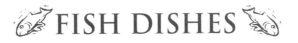

# FISH DISHES

## TARRAGON OVEN-FRIED FISH

### AF (Dairy-free, Egg-free, Corn-free, Gluten-free)

2 pounds fish fillets (sole, snapper, or tilapia)
½ teaspoon salt
1 cup rice thins, crumbled
1 ½ teaspoon tarragon
½ cup milk substitute (soy milk, almond milk, rice milk)
3 tablespoons margarine, melted, dairy-free

Wash and dry fish. Remove any bones. Cut into serving pieces. In small mixing bowl, combine rice crumbs, tarragon, and salt. In separate small bowl, place milk. Dip fish into milk, then into crumb mixture. Place fish into greased 13 by 9 inch baking pan. Cover with remaining crumb mixture. Top with melted margarine. Place in preheated 425 degree oven. Bake for 15 minutes or until the fish flakes easily with fork.
**Serves 6-8**

## CHIPOTLE FISH TACOS

This is a favorite family meal for the summer.

### Testing for Corn (Dairy-free, Egg-free, Gluten-free)

½ cup sorghum flour
1 teaspoon cumin
½ teaspoon chili powder
½ teaspoon garlic powder
½ cup olive oil
1 to 2 pounds white fish (cod, sole, tilapia), cleaned and cut into pieces
2 cups pre-shredded cabbage (can be found in vegetable section of grocery store)
8 to 12 corn tortillas
   Chipotle Dressing *

In flat dish, mix flour and next 3 spices. Brush olive oil onto fish. Coat prepared fish with flour mixture. Place fish into greased baking dish at 400 degrees and bake for 20 minutes, or until fish flakes. A good alternative is to grill the fish for about 20 to 30 minutes. Meanwhile, place corn tortillas in foil. Warm up corn tortillas in oven at 200 degrees. Prepare condiments for taco: tomatoes, onions, olives, dairy-free sour cream, etc. Make Chipotle dressing, recipe below. Mix cabbage with some chipotle dressing. Assemble tacos. First, scoop chipotle dressing into tortilla, then cabbage, add fish and top with condiments.
**Serves 4**

## CHIPOTLE DRESSING*

2 tablespoons chipotle chilies in adobo sauce
½ cup Egg-free mayonnaise

Using vinyl gloves, cut chipotle in half length-wise. Remove seeds from chilies. If you like your sauce HOT, skip this step. Mince chilies and add 1 to 2 tablespoon chilies and at least 2 tablespoons adobo sauce to mayonnaise. Mix to taste and re-frigerate. Can be made up a week in advance.
**Makes ½ cup dressing.**

## TURKEY BACON TROUT

This is a really easy delicious trout recipe

**AF (Dairy-free, Egg-free, Corn-free, Gluten-free)**

4 small to medium trout, dressed
8 strips of turkey bacon
**Marinade:**
$\frac{1}{2}$ cup dry sherry
$\frac{1}{2}$ cup olive oil or melted margarine (corn-free)
2 tablespoons lemon juice
2 tablespoons garlic, minced

Salt the insides of the trout. Mix marinade ingredients: sherry, oil, lemon juice, garlic together in bowl. Place trout in baking dish. Pour marinade over and marinate for 1 to 2 hours. Remove fish from marinade, save left over marinade. Wrap two strip of bacon around each trout. Secure bacon with toothpicks or skewers. Grill over hot heat on barbeque, basting frequently. Grill until bacon is cooked. Turn once.
**Serves 4**

## LINGUINE WITH WHITE CLAM SAUCE

This is my oldest son favorite meal.

### AF (Dairy-free, Egg-free, Corn-free, Gluten-free)

½ cup margarine (corn-free, milk-free)
¼ cup olive oil
1 ¼ cup green onion, chopped
2 (8-ounce) bottles clam juice
2 cloves garlic, minced
2 tablespoons Italian parsley, chopped
2 small tomatoes, chopped
½ teaspoon dried oregano
½ teaspoon dried basil
1/8 teaspoon pepper
2 7-ounce cans of minced clams
One 16 ounce package of rice pasta, either linguine or fettuccini (sometimes difficult to find) may have to use spaghetti rice pasta.*
Romano cheese, shredded (sheep only)

Melt margarine and oil in large skillet over medium heat. Add green onions and saute' until transparent. Add garlic and cook for 30 seconds. Add clam juice, tomatoes, spices, and parsley. Increase heat until boiling, then reduce and simmer for 10 minutes. Add clams and cook another five minutes. Spoon linguine sauce over pasta. Top with Romano shredded cheese.

**Serves 4**

Rice pasta* rice pasta takes longer to cook than regular wheat pasta. Approximately 20 minutes.

**COMPANY HALIBUT**

**AF (Dairy-free, Egg-free, Corn-free, Gluten-free)**

1 ½ pounds fresh halibut
2 tablespoons margarine, corn-free
½ cup onion, chopped
1 garlic clove, minced
¼ cup green peppers, chopped
1 cup celery, sliced
1 cup carrots, sliced thinly
2 sixteen ounce cans diced tomatoes
1 cup Chicken Stock* or Chicken broth
1 teaspoon salt
1 teaspoon thyme
½ teaspoon basil
¼ cup parsley

Cut halibut into 1-inch cubes. In a 12-inch skillet, melt margarine, sauté onion, green pepper, celery and carrots until tender. Add garlic and cook 30 seconds. Add tomatoes, chicken stock, salt and pepper, and spices. Add 2 tablespoons parsley. Bring mixture to boil. Reduce heat, cover and simmer for 25 minutes. Add halibut. Cover and simmer 15 more minutes. Remove halibut from pan, top with sauce. Sprinkle with remaining parsley. Serve mixture over cooked rice.
**Serves 4**

## CHIPOTLE SALMON PATTIES

### Contains Eggs (Dairy-free, Corn-free, Gluten-free)

1 can (15 ½ ounce) salmon
½ cup onion, chopped
¼ cup parsley, chopped
½ cup rice thins, ground
1 egg, beaten
½ teaspoon dried oregano
3 tablespoons oil
Chipotle dressing

Drain and flake salmon, reserving 1/3 cup of liquid. In a large mixing bowl combine salmon, onion, parsley, and ground rice thins. Add beaten egg, oregano, and reserved salmon liquid. Shape into patties. Dry patties with paper towels. Place patties on baking sheet with wax paper. Chill for 30 minutes before cooking. In a large skillet, fry patties in oil until both sides are lightly brown. Serve with Chipotle dressing*(See Dressing and Sauce section) dollop on top of patties. Or if you are out of time prepare a fast version of the Chipotle dressing. To ½ cup mayonnaise or substitute add ½ teaspoon chipotle ground chili pepper, 2 drops of hot sauce, and a dash of cayenne pepper. Mix and chill.
**Served 4**

## SALMON STEAKS WITH TOMATOES

### AF (Dairy-free, Egg-free, Corn-free, Gluten-free) GERD ALERT*

6 salmon steaks
½ cup onions, chopped
1 pound canned tomatoes, finely chopped
4 tablespoons wine vinegar
2 drops Tabasco sauce or Louisiana Hot Sauce
1 teaspoon salt
1 teaspoon white pepper

Place steaks in a large casserole dish. In the microwave, precook onions 30 seconds. In a mixing bowl, mix onions, tomatoes, vinegar, hot sauce, salt and white pepper. Pour mixture over salmon steaks and marinate in refrigerator overnight. Place casserole dish in a moderate 375 degree oven and bake 30 minutes or until tender.
**Serves 6**
        GERD ALERT note: this recipe contain hot sauce and vinegar

## MEXICAN FISH CASSEROLE

### Testing for Dairy (Egg-free, Corn-free, Gluten –free)

1 ½ pounds firm white fish (cod, grouper, sea bass, red snapper)
1 cup sorghum flour
Salt and Pepper
¼ cup margarine, corn-free
8 ounces of fresh or jar red salsa
8 ounces cheddar cheese, shredded
6 ounces jack cheese, shredded
¼ cup parsley, chopped

Preheat oven to 350 degrees. Clean and prepare fish. Cut fish in approximately 3 to 4 inch pieces. Coat fish pieces with flour, salt, and pepper. In 12 inch skillet, melt margarine. Sauté' fish on both sides until lightly brown. Place fish pieces into 9 by 11 baking pan sprayed with pam. Top fish pieces with first 2 tablespoons salsa, then 1to 2 tablespoons cheddar cheese, then 1 teaspoon jack cheese. Place baking pan in oven and bake for 15 minutes or until cheese is melted. Remove from oven. Sprinkle with remaining parsley.
**Serves 6**

## TUNA PATTIES

### AF (Dairy-free, Egg-free**, Corn-free, Gluten-free)

3 tablespoons oil
1 seven-ounce can white albacore tuna, water-packed, drained
¼ cup onion, chopped
½ cup rice thins, ground
2 egg whites
¼ teaspoon dried tarragon
2 tablespoon celery, chopped

Precook celery and onion in microwave 30 seconds. Allow to cool. Combine celery and onion with all the ingredients, shape into patties. In large skillet heat oil and fry each side until lightly brown. Serve on bed of lettuce.
**Serves 2**

## SCALLOPS WITH TOMATO PROVENCE

I like bay scallops for this dish compared to Sea scallops. Sea scallops are a little chewy and not as tender as bay scallops. But bay scallops are more expensive.

### AF (Dairy-free, Egg-free, Corn-free, Gluten-free)

1 pound bay or sea scallops (if using sea scallops, divide each one into fourths)
4 tablespoons olive oil
4 tablespoons sorghum flour
2 fresh garlic cloves, minced
2 tablespoons shallots, finely chopped
½ teaspoon sea salt
1 teaspoon thyme, dried
1 teaspoon basil, dried
½ cup to 1 cup milk substitute (I used plain soy milk)
½ cup dry white wine
¾ cup tomato puree
¼ cup parsley, chopped

Preheat oven to warm, approximately 175 degrees. In large bowl, dredge flour with scallops. In large skillet, add 2 tablespoons oil and heat to medium high. Add scallops and pan fry scallops until brown on all sides. About 7-10 minutes for bay scallops, longer for sea scallops. Remove from skillet, place on plate, cover and keep heated in oven. Add remaining 2 tablespoons oil to skillet; add shallots and sauté until tender. Add garlic and sauté for 30 seconds. Add tomato puree, ¼ cup of the wine, milk substitute, and spices. Simmer for 30 minutes, until thickened. Add more wine or water if sauce becomes too thick.

To assemble: Place a large scoop of sauce on plate. Top sauce with ¼ of scallops and sprinkle with chopped parsley.
**Serves 4**

# ❧ MEAT DISHES ❧
## ❧ BEEF DISHES ❧

**BEEF BURGANDY**

**AF (Dairy-free, Egg-free, Corn-free, Gluten-free)**

2 strips of turkey bacon, sliced
3 tablespoons olive oil
1 onion, sliced
1 package (.54 ounce) of dry porcini mushrooms
1 pound boneless beef chuck roast, cut into ½ inch cubes (can also use stewing meat)
2 cups Burgundy or Pinoir wine
1 ¼ cup beef stock* or beef broth
¼ cup liquid from porcini mushrooms
2 carrots, peeled and chopped
2 garlic cloves, minced
½ cup tomato puree
2 bay leaves
½ teaspoon thyme
½ teaspoon marjoram
¼ teaspoon salt
1/8 pepper

In small bowl place dried porcini mushrooms with 1 cup hot water. Allow to stand for 20 minutes. Drain liquid and mushroom mixture through a sieve. Reserve liquid and chop mushrooms. In large Dutch oven or 9-12 quart pan, place sliced bacon and cook until lightly brown. Remove bacon with slotted spoon (there will not be much fat rendered from turkey bacon). Add 2 tablespoons oil. Add onions and mushrooms and sauté onions until transparent. Remove mushrooms and onions, put in a bowl to the side. Add one more tablespoon of oil. Cut meat into ½ to 1 inch cubes. Sprinkle meat with salt and pepper. Next divide meat in half, cook meat in oil until brown, remove and repeat procedure with other half of cubed meat. Return meat to pan and add mushroom liquid, wine, beef broth, spices, bay leaves, garlic and salt and pepper. Bring to boil, reduce heat and simmer for 1 ½ to 2 hours. When meat is tender, remove bay leaves. Add onion and mushroom mixture with bacon slices. Simmer additional ½ hour more. Thicken with arrowroot. This goes very nicely over rice pasta.
**Serves 6**

## HUNGARIAN GOULASH

**T (Testing for Corn-Dairy-free, Egg-free, Gluten-free)**

2 tablespoon olive oil or grape seed oil
1 ½ pounds chuck pot roast, cut into inch cubes
¼ cup sorghum flour
1 teaspoon salt
½ cup onion, chopped
4 ounces tomato sauce
½ cup beef stock* or beef broth
1 cup water
1 teaspoon paprika
1 bay leaf
1 tablespoon Worcestershire sauce
Dash cayenne
½ cup non-dairy sour cream (most contain corn)
2 tablespoon arrowroot

In flat plate, coat meat with sorghum flour and salt and pepper. In a large skillet with oil heated, brown chuck cubes. Drain any excess oil. Add onion, tomato sauce, beef stock, water, paprika, and bay leaf. Cover and simmer 1 ½ to 2 hours, until beef is tender. Remove bay leaf. Add Worcestershire sauce and then add mixture of non-dairy creamer and arrowroot. Add a dash of cayenne. Do not cook for more than 15 minutes after adding the sour cream.
**Serves 6**

## DAVE'S SPAGHETTI MEAT SAUCE

### AF (Dairy-free, Egg-free, Corn-free, Gluten-free)

2 tablespoons olive oil
1 pound ground beef
2 sixteen-ounce cans tomato sauce
1 medium onion, diced
¼ pound fresh mushrooms, sliced
1 garlic clove, minced
1 tablespoon sugar
3 tablespoons Italian seasoning
1 teaspoon oregano

In large skillet heat oil and brown beef. Drain off grease. Add mushrooms and on-ions, and sauté until onions are transparent. Add remaining ingredients. Cover and simmer for 1 ½ hours. Serve over rice pasta spaghetti or spaghetti squash.
**Serves 4**

## EASY CHILI

### AF (Dairy-free, Egg-free, Corn-free, Gluten-free)

1 pound ground beef, lean
1 medium onion, chopped
1 eight-ounce can tomato sauce
1/3 cup milk substitute (see Appendix A) or Cream of Tomato soup*
1 tablespoon chili powder
1 sixteen-ounce can kidney beans

In large a 12 inch skillet, sauté onion and beef. Drain excess oil. Add tomato sauce and milk substitute (or tomato soup), Chili powder, and kidney beans. Simmer for 45 minutes to 1 hour.
**Serves 4**

## MINCED MEATBALLS

### (Dairy-free, Corn-free, Gluten-free)

1 cup rice thins, ground into crumbs
1 cup milk substitute (See Appendix A)
1 pound lean ground beef
1 egg
$\frac{1}{2}$ teaspoon salt
1/8 teaspoon white pepper
4 tablespoons Manchego or Romano cheese, grated (sheep cheese)
4 tablespoons parsley, finely chopped
1 tablespoon wine vinegar
$\frac{1}{4}$ cup sorghum flour
2 to 3 tablespoons olive oil or grape seed oil

In large mixing bowl, mix first 9 ingredients. Mix and knead mixture to make a paste. Form balls and roll them in flour. Fry meatballs in hot olive oil or grape seed oil until golden.
**Serves 4**

## EGGPLANT AND BEEF

### AF (Dairy-free, Egg-free, Corn-free, Gluten-free)

4 tablespoons margarine, milk-free, corn-free
½ cup celery, sliced
½ cup onion, chopped
¼ cup green pepper, chopped
1 small eggplant, peeled and cubed
2 cups cooked chuck beef, lean
1 eight-ounce can tomato sauce and ¼ cup water
½ teaspoon salt
¼ teaspoon dried marjoram
1/8 teaspoon lemon pepper
1/8 teaspoon ground nutmeg
Dash allspice

Melt margarine in large skillet. Sauté celery, onion and green pepper until tender. Drain off excess margarine. Add eggplant, cooked beef, tomato sauce, water, and spices. Cover and simmer for 45 minutes.
**Serves 8**

**EASY HAMBURGER AND RICE**

I always use this recipe when my boys stomachs were upset.

**(Dairy-free, Egg-free, Gluten-free)**

1 pound ground beef, lean
1 1/2 cups cooked rice
1 cup ketchup, contains corn syrup
½ cup onion, chopped
½ cup water
½ teaspoon salt
Pepper to taste

Brown ground beef and onions together, drain off any grease or liquid. Add ketchup, water, rice and season with salt and pepper. Cook 15 minutes.
**Serves 4**
**Variations:** add mushrooms or cooked green pepper

**STUFFED GREEN PEPPERS**

My Sister likes to use this recipe at Christmas. But she would dye the rice purple.

**AF (Dairy-free, Egg-free, Milk-free, Gluten-free)**

1 pound ground lean beef
½ cup onion, chopped
½ teaspoon salt
1 teaspoon Italian Seasoning
  pepper to taste
1 sixteen ounce tomato sauce
1 ½ cups rice, cooked
4 green peppers

Preheat oven to 400 degrees. In a large skillet, brown beef and onion together. Drain any grease or liquid. Add tomato sauce, seasonings, and simmer for 15 minutes. Add cooked rice to mixture. Cut tops off each pepper; remove seeds and membrane. Blanch peppers in boiling water and rinse with cold water. Drain upside down. Spoon beef and onion mixture into each pepper. Place stuffed peppers in greased casserole dish. Bake in oven for 15 minutes or until pepper are thoroughly heated.
**Served 4**
**Variation:** Top peppers with goat Gouda cheese the last 5 minutes.

## SALISBURY STEAK

### (Dairy-free, Gluten-free)

1 ½ pound ground chuck, lean
½ cup onion, chopped
1 egg, beaten
¼ cup rice thins, ground
½ teaspoon salt
½ teaspoon Italian seasoning
¼ teaspoon turmeric
¼ teaspoon paprika
1 teaspoon onion salt
1 teaspoon garlic salt
Pepper to taste
2 tablespoons vegetable oil or grape seed oil

## WORCESTERSHIRE MUSHRROM SAUCE

½ pound mushrooms, sliced
2 tablespoons margarine (optional)
3 tablespoons sorghum flour
½ cup Beef stock* or beef broth (watch out for maltodextrin which contains corn) ingredient in some soups and broths)
3 tablespoons worcestershire sauce
¼ cup milk or milk substitute*(See Appendix A)

Combine beef, onion, egg, rice thins, and seasonings in bowl. Form mixture in to patties. In large skillet, brown patties. Remove from skillet and set aside. Add margarine to patty dripping, sauté mushrooms until tender. Add sorghum flour to mushrooms; slowly add stock and milk stirring to keep sauce smooth. If sauce seems too thin, add 2 teaspoons arrowroot to 1/3 cup water in separate bowl. Add to sauce and simmer until thickened. Add patties back to skillet. Simmer for 15 to 20 minutes. Serve over rice or rice noodles.
**Serves 6**

## LILIAN'S BEEF JERKY

### AF (Dairy-free, Egg-free, Corn-free, Gluten-free)

1 ½ pound lean beef
1 garlic clove, minced
½ teaspoon salt
Ground pepper
**Marinade:**
Combine in mixing bowl
2 tablespoons miso
2 teaspoons tamari (organic/ wheat-free)
3 tablespoons brown sugar
½ cup canola oil
2 tablespoon red wine vinegar
Alternative Marinade:
Beef Stock*

Rub steak with garlic. In a large casserole, pour marinade over steak. Marinate steak for 24 hours. Pat dry. Trim off fat. Cut strips from meat 1/8 or less in thickness. Cross-grain slices will be more tender than with- grain trips. Add salt and pepper to strips.

Place strips on rack of a baking pan. Bake in a preheated 150 degree oven for 4 hours. Prop oven door open at tip approximately 3-6 inches. Turn strips several times during drying process. Test for dryness. Store jerky in covered jars in cool, dry place in refrigerator.

**Makes approximately 25 pieces**
Note: with new drying stoves, part two of this recipe is not needed. Instead follow instructions of the stove.

## MARINATED FLANK STEAK

### AF (Dairy-free, Egg-free, Corn-free, Gluten-free)

1 ½ pounds flank steak
**Marinade:**
2 teaspoons tamari soy sauce (organic/wheat-free)
2 tablespoons miso
3 tablespoons brown sugar
2 tablespoons red vinegar
1 garlic clove, minced
½ cup canola oil
2 shallots, sliced
1 teaspoon ground ginger

In mixing bowl, combine marinade ingredients. Pour over steak. Marinate overnight in refrigerator. When ready to cook, pat meat dry and place on a cooking sheet. Place under broiler for 3 -5 minutes. Slice diagonally and serve.
**Serves 4-6**

## ORIENTAL PEPPER STEAK

### AF (Dairy-free, Egg-free, Corn-free, Gluten-free)

1 ½ pounds round steak
3 tablespoons canola oil
1 cup onion, sliced
1 pound canned tomatoes
1 teaspoon salt
½ teaspoon white pepper
2 bay leaves
2 large green peppers, seeded and cut into strips
2 tablespoons arrowroot
2 teaspoons tamari soy sauce (organic/ wheat-free)
¼ cup cold water
Parsley

Cut round steak into ¼ inch-wide strips. In a large skillet, heat oil, and brown meat strips quickly on both sides. Remove from skillet and set aside. Add onions and sauté until tender. Add tomatoes with liquid, salt, pepper, and bay leaves. Cover and simmer for 45 minutes to 1 hour. Stir in green peppers. Continue cooking for 15 minutes longer.

In separate mixing bowl, blend arrowroot, tamari and cold water, and add mixture to skillet. Cook until thickened, about 1 minute. Serve over a bed of rice. Garnish with parsley.
**Serves 6**

# LAMB DISHES

Lamb is a wonderful meat and is known is cause little allergy problems. What people don't like about lamb is its gamy taste. The trick to lamb so that taste doesn't happen is to sear the meat first before cooking. In all the following recipes, I will do searing almost every time. Special note: using non-stick pans for high heat unless it specifically states it can handle high heat, is not a good idea.

## DON'S BAREQUED LEG OF LAMB

My cousin's husband has this wonderful recipe for barbecued lamb. I had to change Don's recipe a little bit to make it allergy-free.

### AF (Dairy-free, Egg-free, Corn-free, Gluten-free)

5 to 8 pound butterfly leg of lamb, with most fat removed, some left for flavor
½ cup Organic Tamari Sauce (Naturally brewed)
¼ cup of Hoisin sauce
½ cup extra virgin olive oil
1 cup sweet wine (rose, blush or white Grenache jug wine)
6 to 8 large garlic cloves, pressed
2 tablespoons Fresh rosemary leaves, finely chopped
1 tablespoon thyme, dried
1 tablespoon marjoram, dried
Zest of one lemon, plus, rest of lemon cut into quarters

Mix marinate together in bowl, marinate lamb in bag or baking dish for 8 to 24 hours. Save marinate for grilling. Preheat Grill. Cook lamb on high to medium high. Start with the lamb fat side up. Turn every 7-10 minutes applying marinate as needed. Grill until the internal temperature at the thickest point is 130, higher if you like your lamb well done. Take off grill and let rest. The temperature of the lamb will rise while it is resting. Slice and serve.
**Serves 8 to 10**

## BASIC LAMB STEW

### AF (Dairy-free, Egg-free, Corn-free, Gluten-free)

2 tablespoon grape seed oil (good for high heat cooking)
2 ½ pounds lamb, cut into 1-inch cubes
½ cup onion, chopped
1 cup water or beef broth or Beef Stock*
2 cups tomatoes, chopped
2 cups potatoes, sliced
   salt and pepper to taste

In large skillet, heat oil to medium-high. Sear lamb until brown. Remove lamb to a plate and set aside. Add more oil if needed and sauté onions until tender. Add lamb and liquid and simmer for 1 hour. Add tomatoes, potatoes, salt, and pepper. Cover and simmer for 45 minutes or until potatoes are tender.
**Serves 8**

## FRENCH ONION BAKED LAMB CHOPS

### T (Testing for milk—Egg-free, Corn-free, Gluten-free)

4 thick lamb chops
1 cup sour cream
2 tablespoon sorghum flour
1 cup French Onion Soup*thickened with arrowroot
2 tablespoons parsley, chopped

In a 9 by 13-inch casserole dish or baking pan, place lamb chops under a hot broiler and brown for 8-10-minutes on each side( depending on thickness). In a mixing bowl, combine flour and sour cream. Add French Onion soup and parsley. Pour mixture over lamb chops and cover. Bake at 350 degrees for one hour.
**Serves 4**

## LAMB CHOPS WITH TARRAGON

### AF (Dairy-free, Egg-free, Corn-free, Gluten-free)

4 lamb chops
1 tablespoon grape seed oil
½ cup carrots, peeled and sliced
½ cup celery, chopped
1 cup onion, chopped
1 garlic clove, minced
2 tablespoons margarine, corn-free
¼ teaspoon tarragon wine vinegar
½ cup Beef broth or Beef Stock*
1 teaspoon tarragon
   salt and pepper to taste

Rub lamb chops with minced garlic clove. In a large skillet on high heat add grape seed oil. Sear lamb chops on both sides until meat is pink. Remove to plate and set aside. Reduce heat to medium. Add 2 tablespoon margarine to skillet, sauté onion, carrots, and celery until onion is transparent and carrot tender. Add lamb chops, beef stock, vinegar, tarragon and salt and pepper. Bring to boil, reduce heat, cover and simmer until lamb is done, approximately 20 minutes.
**Serves 4**

## LAMB AND LIMA BEANS

### AF (Dairy-free, Egg-free, Corn-free, Gluten-free)

6 tablespoon margarine, milk-free, corn-free
1 ½ pounds lamb shoulder, cut into 1-inch cubes
4 small onions, sliced
2 packages frozen lima beans
½ cup sliced mushrooms
6 fresh tomatoes, quartered, or 1 sixteen ounce can tomatoes
½ cup water
   salt and pepper

In large skillet, melt 4 tablespoons of the margarine over high heat. (If the margarine is smoking, your heat is too high.) Quickly sear lamb meat until brown and meat is just pink. Remove lamb; set aside. Keep warm. Melt remaining margarine with lamb drippings, and add onions and mushrooms; sauté until tender. Add lima beans, tomatoes, water, salt and pepper. Simmer until thickened. Return lamb to mixture and cook until meat is heated through, approximately 20 minutes. Serve over rice.
**Serves 4-6**

## STUFFED CABBAGGE ROLLS

### AF (Dairy-free, Egg-free, Corn-free, Gluten-free)

¾ cup uncooked rice, rinsed in cold water
1 ½ pound coarsely ground lamb
½ teaspoon salt
1/8 teaspoon pepper
Dash of allspice
Dash of nutmeg
1 head of cabbage, boiled until just limp
2 garlic cloves, chopped
1 sixteen ounce can tomatoes, diced
Water if necessary

Preheat oven to 350 degrees. In a medium-size bowl, mix rice, ground lamb, salt, pepper, allspice, and nutmeg. Place a small amount of meat mixture on each cooked cabbage leaf and roll. Place rolls in Dutch oven. Sprinkle chopped garlic between rolls. Pour tomatoes with juice over cabbage rolls. Add just enough water to cover rolls, if necessary. Bake at 350 degrees for 20 minutes.
**Serves 6**

## LAMB CURRY

Make sure you have really good curry for this recipe. Bland curry takes away from the taste. I added some Crushed Red Peppers to give it a little zip.

### AF (Dairy-free, Egg-free, Corn-free, Gluten-free)

1 ½ pound lamb, (shoulder or pieces cut from leg) cut into 1 to 1 ½ inch cubes
1 cup onion, chopped
¼ cup green pepper, chopped
¼ cup celery, chopped
2 garlic cloves, minced
2 tablespoons grape seed oil (good for high heat cooking) or vegetable oil
2 teaspoons curry powder
½ teaspoon salt
¼ cup sorghum flour
3 cups Chicken stock* or chicken broth
2 tablespoons arrowroot in ¼ cup water for thickening

In large skillet, heat grape seed oil over high to medium-high heat. Add lamb. Sear meat until pink. Reduce heat. Remove meat from pan with slotted spoon. Set aside. Cook in lamb drippings the onion, green peppers, celery and garlic. Sauté vegetables until onions are transparent. Add flour, salt and curry to pan. Slowly add chicken broth to mixture to aviod any lumps. Return lamb to skillet. Cover and simmer for 45 minutes or until lamb is tender. Serve over brown or white Basmati rice.
**Serves 6**

# PORK DISHES

Pork is known to cause problems involving the digestion system. Mostly, those symptoms are caused by the fatty cuts of pork: Ham, and bacon. The lean sections of the pig are not as troublesome. In this section I will test for problems with pork with lean meat cuts.

## SOUTHWESTERN POZOLE STEW

**T (Testing for pork—Dairy-free, Egg-free, Gluten-free)**

1 ½ pounds pork, shoulder cut with bone in. 3 pounds with bone in yields about 1 to ½ pounds. Keep bone, just one large one.
2 tablespoons grape seed oil, or canola oil
1 cup onions, chopped
2 garlic cloves, minced
1 (14.5 ounce) can tomatoes, diced
1 (7.5 ounce) can green chilies, diced
2 medium size carrots, peeled and sliced
4 cups Chicken stock* or chicken broth
1 (14.5 ounce) can white or yellow hominy,
   drained and rinsed (hominy is a corn product)
¼ cup cilantro, chopped

In large saucepan (approximately 5 quart size) add oil, sauté onions until they are transparent. Add pork cubes, garlic and brown until pork is no longer pink. Take care not to burn meat. Remove pork from pan and set aside. Add chicken broth, tomatoes, green chilies, spices, bone and bring to boil. Add pork mixture into sauce pan and reduce heat. Simmer without cover, for about 45 minutes or until liquid is reduced about 1 inch. Add hominy and cilantro; cover and simmer for another 45 minutes or until pork meat is tender and shreds easily. Remove bone with slotted spoon. Serve in soup bowl with heated corn tortillas.
**Serves 6**

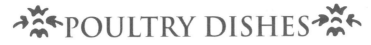

# POULTRY DISHES

Before cooking chicken, or turkey it is worth the extra step to brine the meat pieces. Brining usually takes 24 hours for a whole bird, less for chicken pieces. There are some quick ways to brine if you are in a hurry. Brining instructions are at the end of this section.

## CHICKEN DISHES

### CHICKEN CACCIATORE

**AF (Dairy-free, Egg-free, Corn-free, Gluten-free)**

¼ cup olive oil
1 frying chicken (2 ½ to 3 pounds), cut into serving pieces
1 onion, chopped
2 garlic cloves, minced (can use commercial crushed garlic instead, use 2 tablespoons)
1 cup Chicken stock* or chicken broth
1 (14.5 ounce) can whole tomatoes
1 (6 ounce) can tomato paste
½ cup wine, white
½ teaspoon thyme leaves
2 bay leaves
1 teaspoon salt (If the chicken was brined first, omit salt. In this recipe the chicken does not need to be brined.)
½ teaspoon pepper
Dash crushed red peppers (careful not too much)

Wash chicken pieces and pat dry with paper towels. Place oil in large skillet, 12 inch or larger. Heat oil, add chicken and brown slightly. Remove chicken to plate and set aside. Add onion and garlic, sauté until onion is transparent. Drain any excess grease or liquid. Return chicken to skillet. Add broth, tomatoes, tomato paste, wine, spices and salt and pepper. Cover and simmer for 1 to 1½ hours. Uncover and cook another ½ hour. Serve chicken over rice.

**Serves 6**

Note: My oldest son never liked mushrooms, so I never put mushrooms in this dish. It was easier than watching him pick them all out. However, if you would like to add mushrooms, add ½ cup sliced Crimini mushroom with the onions and garlic. You may need more oil.

## CHICKEN AND CHIPOTLE SAUCE BURITTOS

### T (Testing for corn—Dairy-free, Egg-free, Gluten-free)

2 tablespoons olive oil or canola oil
1 cup onion, chopped
1 garlic clove, minced
2 cups cooked chicken, chopped or shredded
2 small chipotle peppers in adobo sauce, minced (Be sure to wear vinyl gloves when chopping the peppers. If you do not want it too hot, remove the seeds inside the chilies. Save the rest of the chipotle peppers and sauce to make chipotle dressing. Recipe is in Dressing and Sauces section.)
1 ½ tablespoons black olives, chopped
1 cup tomato sauce
½ cup water
¾ teaspoon oregano
½ teaspoon cumin
Salt and Pepper to taste

In large sauce pan, heat oil. Add onion and garlic then sauté until onions are transparent. Add tomato sauce, oregano, cumin, chopped chicken, chipotle peppers, olives, salt and pepper. Simmer for 15 minutes. Watch thickness. You may need to add water. Use this sauce as a filling for corn tortillas. The tortillas need to be fresh. Warm the tortillas up by putting in wet cloth, placing on plate and putting in warm oven. Add condiments such as: fresh chopped cilantro; goat Colby cheese, shredded; sour cream (milk substitute-contains soy and some also contain maltodextrin).
**Serves 4**

## SNAPPY OVEN FRIED CHICKEN AND STUFFING

### AF (Dairy-free, Egg-free, Corn-free, Gluten-free)

1 ½ cubes hard margarine or 12 tablespoons soft margarine (corn-free, milk-free)
3 pound fryer chicken, cut in to pieces (save the giblets), try to remove most of the skin
¾ cup sorghum flour
¼ cup amaranth flour
½ teaspoon salt
¼ teaspoon pepper
1/8 teaspoon cayenne pepper
1/8 teaspoon red pepper chilies (optional)

Preheat oven to 425 degrees. In 9 by 13 inch baking pan and in an 8 by 8 inch baking pan, melt margarine. Meanwhile, mix flours, spices, and salt and pepper together. Wash chicken and place on paper towels. Dredge chicken in flour mixture and lay meat side down in pan. Bake at 425 uncovered for 30 minutes. Remove from oven and turn chicken pieces. Return to oven for 30 minutes more or until the juices of the chicken run clear. Serve with Chicken Stuffing (recipe to follow) and Chicken gravy found in Dressing and Sauces Section.
**Serves 6**

## SAVORY CHICKEN STUFFING

### AF (Dairy-free, Egg-free*, Corn-free, Gluten-free)

1 homemade, day old, gluten-free bread, crust removed, cubed. Store bought gluten-free bread cannot be frozen. It is too heavy to make decent stuffing
3 tablespoon canola oil
1 cup celery, chopped
1 cup onion, chopped
³/₄ to 1 cup Chicken stock* or chicken broth
2 tablespoon margarine, melted, dairy-free, corn-free
1 teaspoon poultry seasoning
1 teaspoon sage
¹/₂ teaspoon salt
¹/₄ teaspoon pepper

Slice bread and let it dry out for 2 hours. Cut bread into cubes and put into bowl. In saucepan, place oil and heat. Add onion and celery, sauté 3 to 4 minutes or until onions are transparent. Cool slightly and add to bread cubes. Add liquids, margarine and spices. Mix together and put into 2 quart casserole dish, cover. Bake for 30 minutes at 350 degrees. Uncover and cook for another 10 minutes. Serve with gravy and chicken.

**Serves 6**

Note: If the oven is being used put casserole in microwave for 10 minutes. Then put into oven uncovered for 15 minutes at 375 degrees or until stuffing is light brown.

## CHICKEN AND TURKEY SAUSAGE GUMBO

### AF (Dairy-free, Egg-free, Corn-free, Gluten-free)

1 ½ teaspoons salt
1 ½ teaspoons black pepper
1 teaspoon red pepper (cayenne)
1 teaspoon white pepper
1 three pound chicken fryer, cut into pieces
½ cup white rice flour
½ cup canola oil
2 large onions, finely chopped
2 bell peppers, finely chopped
1 cup celery, finely chopped
4 to 5 cups chicken broth, heated
1 pound turkey sausage, sliced ½ inch thick
¾ cup green onion, chopped
¾ cup parsley, chopped
¼ teaspoon Louisiana hot sauce
2 tablespoons margarine, dairy-free, corn-free

Clean chicken, pat dry on paper towels. Place chicken on plate. In small bowl, mix salt, red, white, and black peppers. Sprinkle pepper mixture over chicken pieces. In 5 to 9 quart Dutch oven heat oil to high heat. Stir rice flour into oil. Stir constantly until flour mixture turns brown this will take about 20 minutes. This can be labor intensive, have a friend or spouse to this while you are cooking the vegetables. Meanwhile, in large skillet heat margarine, add green peppers and sauté 1 minute by itself. Then add onions and celery. You may need more margarine. Finish sautéing the onions, celery, and green peppers until tender. Transfer onions, celery and pepper to Dutch oven. Next add heated chicken broth to Dutch oven by stirring slowly into flour roux to avoid any lumps. Add rest of pepper and salt mixture. Bring to a boil. Let simmer for 45 minutes.

Back to the skillet, cook turkey sausage, in skillet until brown. Add to Dutch oven. Add additional oil to skillet if needed. Add chicken and brown on each side, transfer to Dutch oven. Simmer for another 1½ hours until chicken is tender. Remove Dutch oven from heat. Stir in green onion, parsley, and hot sauce. Let sit a few minutes. Serve over rice.

**Serves 6-8**

## CHICKEN STEW

### AF (Dairy-free, Egg-free, Corn-free, Gluten-free)

2 tablespoons margarine, dairy-free, corn-free
1 stewing chicken, cut into pieces
1 sixteen-ounce can tomatoes, diced, (save liquid)
½ Chicken Stock* or chicken broth
1 teaspoon salt
3 peppercorns
1 sixteen-ounce can garbanzo beans
½ cup almonds, sliced
½ cup water, boiling

In large skillet melt margarine, add chicken and brown on both sides until golden. Remove chicken and set aside. Add onion and sauté until tender. Return chicken to skillet. Add tomatoes, chicken stock, salt, peppercorns, and enough liquid from canned tomatoes to cover. Simmer chicken mixture for 1 hour. Mix garbanzo beans with remaining tomato liquid or a little boiling water and add to chicken. Mix well. Stir in almonds and cook for 10 minutes more. Serve hot in bowls.
**Serves 8**

## CHICKEN MARSALA

### (Dairy-free, Corn-free, Gluten-free)

4 chicken breasts, skinned and brined
1 egg or egg substitute, beaten
¼ cup sorghum flour
3 tablespoon olive oil
2 cups Crimin mushrooms, sliced
1 cup Marsala
1 tablespoon parsley, chopped
¼ teaspoon salt
1/8 teaspoon pepper

Clean chicken pieces, pat dry on paper towels. Dip chicken breasts in egg in bowl, and then in flour. In large skillet, heat oil over medium-high heat. Brown the chicken

on both sides. Remove chicken to a plate and set aside. Leave drippings in skillet. Add 1 teaspoon oil to skillet. Add the mushrooms to the skillet and sauté until tender about 4 minutes. Return chicken to skillet. Add Marsala, parsley and salt and pepper. Heat mixture until hot about 10 to 15 minutes. If sauce is to thin, add 1 tablespoon arrowroot mixed with 1/8 cup of water to the sauce. Serve over rice pasta.
**Serves 4**

## CHICKEN A LA KING

**T (Testing for gluten—Dairy-free, Egg-free, Corn-free)**

2 cups chicken, cooked and cubed
3 tablespoons margarine, dairy-free, corn-free
½ cup all-purpose flour
1 ½ cups milk substitute
½ cup Chicken Stock* or chicken broth
¼ cup shallots, sliced
½ cup fresh mushrooms, sliced
¼ cup green pepper, chopped
1 four ounce jar pimento, drained, chopped
1 teaspoon salt
¼ teaspoon pepper

Melt margarine in a skillet. Add shallots and green peppers, sauté until tender. Add flour and stir until well blended. Slowly add milk substitute and chicken stock. Add chicken, mushrooms, pimento, salt and pepper. Simmer over medium heat for 15 minutes. Serve over toast.
**Serves 4-6**

## CHINESE CHICKEN BREASTS

This is one of those easy dinners to fix and it is so good for you. Buy packaged cooked chicken and veggies at the store. Make rice in rice cooker while chopping vegetables and cooking. This meal is easy and fast.

### AF (Dairy-free, Egg-free, Corn-free, Gluten-free)

1 ½ pounds chicken breasts, boneless, cooked
(grilled packaged precooked chicken works well)
2 tablespoons sesame seed oil
2 tablespoons arrowroot
¼ cup water
1 tablespoon tamari soy sauce (traditional/wheat-free/gluten-free)
2 teaspoons commercial crushed garlic (I like Trader Joe's)
1 cup onion, chopped
¼ cup shallots, sliced
½ cup green pepper, chopped
1 cup snow peas, ends cut off and sliced in half
½ cup mushrooms, sliced
1 can water chestnuts (optional)
2 cups bean sprouts
½ blanched almonds
¼ teaspoon salt
1/8 teaspoon pepper

Slice cooked chicken into small pieces. Heat chicken pieces in large skillet with some oil. Remove chicken from skillet. Add celery, onions, and sauté until tender. Add green pepper, peas, mushrooms, water chestnuts, bean sprouts, almonds, salt, and pepper. Cook until vegetables are chewy but not tender. Return chicken to skillet. Heat.

In small mixing bowl, mix arrowroot, water and tamari. Cook over medium heat until thoroughly heated and thickened. Pour over vegetables and chicken. Serve with rice.
**Serves 4**

## SPINACH CHICKEN BREASTS

### AF (Dairy-free, Egg-free, Corn-free, Gluten-free)

3 tablespoons olive oil
6 chicken breasts, boneless, skinless
¼ cup shallots, chopped
½ cup sorghum flour
1 package spinach, fresh
1 tablespoon fresh dill, chopped or ½ teaspoon dried dill
2 tablespoons fennel, chopped
¼ teaspoon salt
1/8 teaspoon pepper
1/8 teaspoon nutmeg
2 to 3 ounces Feta cheese, crumbled (imported/goat)
1 cup hot Chicken stock* or chicken broth

Clean and dry chicken breasts. Pound chicken until ½ to ¼ inch thick. Dip each breast into flour mixture, and brown in a large skillet in hot oil. Remove chicken and set aside on warm platter. Reduce heat. Add shallots and fennel, sauté until tender. Wash and clean spinach (you can skip this step if you have cleaned prepared spinach). Chop spinach and add to shallots in skillet. Add rest of the ingredients: dill, fennel, salt , pepper, and nutmeg. Place chicken breasts in 13 by 9 baking dish, and spoon spinach mixture over breasts. Place Feta cheese on top of spinach mixture, and pour hot chicken stock or broth over all. Place in a 375 degree oven and bake until Feta is softened, about 40 minutes.
**Serves 4**

## BARBECUED CHICKEN

Everyone has their special way to barbecue chicken, this is just one way.

### AF (Dairy-free, Egg-free, Corn-free, Gluten-free)

2 ½-3 pound cut up chicken
3 cups Spicy Barbecue Sauce*
Salt and pepper

Brine chicken pieces 24 hours before grilling. Dry chicken pieces on paper towels. Preheat gas grill or charcoal barbecue. Grease grill rack. Season chicken with salt and pepper. Place dark meat first on the barbecue, cooking with skin side down. Then add white meat (during the AF dieting only white meat is supposed to be used). Over medium direct heat, cook for 5 minutes on one side. Turn chicken as needed basting with barbecue sauce. Continue to cook chicken 10 to 15 minutes or until juices run clear.

**Serves 4**

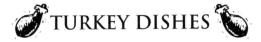

# TURKEY DISHES

## TURKEY GOULASH

**T (Testing for milk—Egg-free, Corn-free, Gluten-free)**

2 tablespoons oil, canola or grape seed
3 cups turkey, cooked and chopped
1 cup onion, chopped
1 garlic clove, minced
1 ¾ cup Chicken Stock*or chicken broth
1 cup tomato sauce
1 tablespoon paprika
1 teaspoon salt
½ teaspoon pepper
1 cup sour cream

Add oil to large skillet, add onions and garlic. Sauté onions and garlic. Add turkey, stock, tomato sauce, and seasonings. Simmer for 20 to 30 minutes. Remove from heat and stir in sour cream. Serve over rice or rice pasta.

**Serves 6**

Note: By using milk substitute sour cream this recipe can become a AF recipe. However most substitute sour creams contain soy or corn starch.

## TURKEY/SAUSAGE LOAF

There is a variety of moisture content between ground turkey meats. The" Trader Joe" variety is very moist and needs more bread crumbs than other brands. Special note: I love to chop. It relaxes me. But many individuals will not agree with that. So an easy way to get past the chopping on the onions, carrots, and celery is put them in a food processor for 5 pulses. I like to call these vegetables the "three amigos" because I use them together so often.

**(Dairy-free, Corn-free, Gluten-free)**

1 pound turkey, ground
½ pound sausage turkey, casings removed
2 tablespoons olive oil
½ cup onion, chopped
1 celery stalk, finely chopped
1 carrot, peeled and shredded
2 tablespoons hard goat or sheep cheese, grated
(I like Gouda goat or Manchego sheep)
2 tablespoons Italian parsley, chopped
1 garlic clove, minced
¾ teaspoon salt
¼ teaspoon pepper
1 teaspoon oregano
1 tablespoon Worcestershire sauce
½ cup rice bread crumb or ground rice thins
2 tablespoons tomato paste
2 tablespoons water
1 egg beaten
2 slices of turkey bacon

In large skillet, sauté onions, celery, and carrots in oil until tender. Cool. In large bowl, combine ground turkey, turkey sausage, cheese, parsley, garlic, Worcestershire, spices, bread crumbs, tomato paste and water mixed, and egg. Add cooked onion mixture. Mix together and form 2 loafs. Place into greased 8 by 8 inch baking dish. Cut bacon strips to fit loaves and then in half vertically. Place bacon strips horizontally across the loaves, 4 on each loaf. Bake at 350 degrees for 1 hour.
**Serves 4**

## TURKEY DIVAN

### T (Testing for gluten—Dairy-free, Egg-free, Corn-free)

2 cups of left -over turkey in slices, or ¼ inch thick slices of commercial turkey
½ pound of fresh broccoli, steamed OR 2 packages of frozen broccoli,
    thawed and patted dry
2 teaspoons margarine, milk-free, corn-free
½ cup water
½ cup onion, chopped
2 tablespoons flour
1 ¾ cups Cream of Mushroom soup (if you want lots of gluten,
    Campells is the brand to choose)
½ teaspoon salt
¾ teaspoon curry
½ to 1 cup soft wheat bread crumbs
2 teaspoons margarine, melted, milk-free, corn-free

Prepare turkey slices and set aside. In small skillet or saucepan, melt margarine. Add onions and sauté until tender. Add flour, water, salt, and cream of mushroom soup. Heat until slightly thickened, add curry powder.

Place broccoli in greased 9 by 13 baking dish. Layer sliced cooked turkey on top. Pour heated sauce over broccoli and turkey. Sprinkle with breadcrumbs and pour melted margarine over all. Bake covered in a preheated oven of 375 degrees for 30 to 35 minutes.
**Serves 4 to 6**

An AF-Diet version of this recipe changes the following: Use 1 tablespoon sorghum flour instead of regular flour. The cream of mushroom soup must be organic or Progresso. There are some great mushroom soups out there. Try Walnut acres Organic Creamy Portabella mushroom soup. Check the label for wheat sources or milk sources. Use the rice flour bread from Ener-g for the breadcrumbs and margarine for the butter.

## TURKEY TETRAZZINI

### AF (Dairy-free, Egg-free, Corn-free, Gluten-free)

¼ cup margarine, dairy-free, corn-free
1 pound mushrooms, sliced
½ cup onions, chopped
1 tablespoon lemon juice
1 teaspoon salt
1 teaspoon paprika
¼ cup sorghum flour
1 ¾ cup Chicken Stock* or Chicken broth
½ cup milk substitute
3 cups turkey, cubed
1 (8 ounce package) rice pasta, cooked

Melt margarine in a skillet. Sauté mushrooms and onions. Stir in flour; slowly add milk, stock, and seasonings. Simmer for 15 minutes, add turkey. Place cooked pasta in a greased 1 ½ quart casserole. Pour turkey mixture over rice pasta, and bake for 20 minutes at 350 degrees. If the sauce is not thickened, add in small bowl, 2 teaspoons arrowroot to 1/3 cup water. Mix together and add to sauce. Simmer to thicken.
**Serves 4**

## HOT TURKEY SANDWICHES

### AF (Dairy-free, Egg-free**, Corn-free, Gluten-free)

1 pound Roasted Turkey, (wheat-free, ask at you meat counter)
Homemade gluten-free bread or commercial rice bread (not frozen)
Turkey/ Chicken gravy*(recipe to follow)

Heat turkey slices. Oven toast bread slices (especially rice bread). Place meat slices on bread slices. Pour gravy over. Serve hot.
**Serves 4**

## TURKEY GIBLET/CHICKEN GRAVY

### AF (Dairy-free, Egg-free, Corn-free, Gluten-free)

$\frac{1}{2}$ cup onion, finely chopped
$\frac{1}{2}$ cup celery, finely chopped
3 tablespoons giblets, chopped (if possible)
4 tablespoons margarine, dairy-free
$\frac{1}{4}$ cup plus 1 tablespoon white rice flour
1 cup beef broth (for color)
3 cups chicken broth
2 bay leaves
$\frac{1}{2}$ teaspoon poultry seasoning
$\frac{1}{2}$ teaspoon sage
$\frac{1}{2}$ teaspoon salt
$\frac{1}{4}$ teaspoon pepper
1 tablespoon arrowroot mixed with 1/8 cup water to thicken

In large saucepan, heat margarine until melted. Add giblets, onion, celery, and sauté for about 5 minutes. Add 1 tablespoon flour and stir to make roux. Gradually add broth, stirring so not to cause lumps. Add to sauce spices, salt and pepper and bay leaves. Simmer until 1 inch of the liquid is evaporated. Then cover and simmer another 20 minutes. Strain gravy through meshed sieve into another sauce pan. Add 2 tablespoons arrowroot dissolved in $\frac{1}{4}$ cup water to thicken.
**Makes 4 cups**

# TURKEY BURGER WITH ASIAN CRANBERRY SAUCE

## AF (Dairy-free, Egg-free**, Corn-free, Gluten-free)

1 pound turkey, ground, dark meat
1 cup rice bread crumbs or rice thins ground
$\frac{1}{2}$ cup celery, chopped
1/3 cup shallots, finely chopped
2 tablespoons margarine, corn-free, milk-free
1 teaspoon thyme
$\frac{1}{2}$ teaspoon sage
$\frac{1}{2}$ teaspoon salt
$\frac{1}{4}$ teaspoon pepper
2 tablespoons parsley, chopped
1 egg beaten or 2 egg whites beaten
Dave's Asian Cranberry Sauce*

In large skillet, heat margarine then sauté celery and shallots. Cook until transparent. Allow to cool. In large bowl, Mix all ingredients together and form into patties. Grill each burger 4 to 6 minutes on each side. Place on lettuce or toasted rice bread. Top with Dave's Asian Cranberry sauce.
**Makes 4-6 patties**

**Dave's Asian Cranberry Sauce***
1 package dried cranberries
2 cups water
1 tablespoon Hoisin sauce
1 teaspoon Chinese 5 spice
2 tablespoons orange juice

Place dried cranberries in saucepan with water. Heat to boiling, boil for 5 minutes and cool. Drain cramberries through a sieve. Place cranberries in to food processor, add remaining ingredients. Process together. Chill. Return to room temperature before turkey burgers are grilled. Sauce can be made 2 days ahead. **Makes 1 $\frac{1}{4}$ cup of sauce**

## TURKEY BACON AND CHEESE SANDWICH

### AF (Dairy-free, Egg-free, Corn-free, Gluten-free)

8 slices commercial rice bread, not frozen (Ener-g is AF safe)
16 slices of turkey bacon, cut in half and cooked
8 (¼ to ½ inch thick) slices jalapeno jack cheese, goat
½ to 1 cup olive oil
3 cups cilantro, washed, stems removed

With olive oil, brush each bread slice on one side. Place 4 half pieces of the cooked bacon on slices. Place cheese and cilantro on slices. Cover each prepared bread with other bread slices. Brush oil on outside of bread slices so all sides are now brushed with oil. Place on hot skillet and cook on each side until golden brown and cheese is melted. Serve immediately.
**Serves 4**

## TURKEY BACON LETTUCE AND TOMATO SANDWICH
This recipe does not work on frozen gluten-free bread.

### AF (Dairy-free, Egg-free, Corn-free, Gluten-free)

1 tablespoon olive oil
8 slices turkey bacon, cut in half
½ cup flavored olive oil (I used basil flavor)
4 sliced Gluten-free bread (my husband likes the tapioca flour)
2 tomatoes, sliced
½ - 1 cup imitation mayonnaise (i.e. Vegenaise)
1 teaspoon wholegrain champagne mustard
Butter lettuce

In large skillet, heat olive oil, add turkey pieces and cook on each side for about 2 minutes until done. Remove from skillet and drain on paper towels. Wash and dry lettuce, and slice tomatoes. In small bowl, mix imitation mayonnaise and mustard. Reheat large skillet, add 2 tablespoon of flavored olive oil. Add bread and fry on both sides, adding more olive oil as needed. This bread is very thick and needs more oil than wheat breads. Assemble by first spreading mayonnaise mixture on bread slices. Then add 2 turkey slices, tomato and lettuce.
**Makes 4 sandwiches.**

## BRINING INSTRUCTIONS

Because most of the meat cuts we are using are lean or range fed, many of these meats and poultry will not be as tender as we are used to. Also many types of meat, especially chicken, need to be brined before grilling. We need to increase the water retention of the meat before we cook it. The best candidates for brining are: turkey, chicken, pork and some fishes.

Salt, sugar, and water are the three ingredients necessary for brining. Table salt can be used for short periods, but kosher salt is better and less salty.

1. Large cuts of meat: 1 gallon of water to 1 cup kosher salt to 1 cup of sugar. In large container mix water, salt, and sugar. Dissolve salt and sugar thoroughly. Place meat into container, cover for 12 to 24 hours. Remove from container and pat dry. Let meat dry in refrigerator to allow surface moisture to evaporate. Diamond brand kosher salt seems to work the best.

2. Small cuts of meat: 1 quart container (I sometimes use plastic bags) to ¼ cup kosher salt to ¼ cup sugar. Follow same instructions as above. If using table salt cut the amount in half.

# 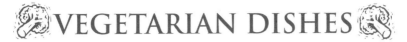VEGETARIAN DISHES

**VEGETABLE SHEPERD PIE**

This is a great meal to have with leftover mash potatoes. The package mash potatoes have corn starch in them.

**AF (Dairy-free, Egg-free, Corn-free, Gluten-free)**

2 tablespoons olive oil
1 cup onion, chopped
¾ cup celery, sliced
1 ¼ cup carrots, peeled and coarsely chopped
1 cup turnip, peeled and coarsely chopped
2 garlic cloves, minces
2 cups vegetable broth
1 (14.5 ounce) can tomatoes, diced
2 bay leaves
1 ½ teaspoon thyme
1 teaspoon basil
½ teaspoon salt
Pepper to taste
1 (15 ounces) cannellini white beans, drained
1 portabella mushroom cap, stem removed, coarsely chopped
1 zucchini, sliced

**Mash Potatoes:**
5 medium potatoes, peeled, cubed, and cooked
2 tablespoons milk Substitute
1 tablespoon margarine

Cook and mash potatoes with milk and margarine before starting vegetables. Set aside. In large skillet/ saucepan, heat oil. Add carrots, onions and celery, sauté until the onions are transparent. Add broth, tomatoes, garlic, turnip, bay leaves, spices, salt and pepper. Bring mixture to boil. Reduce until simmer. Cook vegetables and broth for 45 minutes to 60 minutes or until veggies are just tender. Remove bay leaves. Add mushrooms, beans and zucchini. Place in large baking dish or casserole dish. Spread the mash potatoes on top of vegetable mixture. Cook at 350 degrees for 20 minutes or until golden brown.

**Serves 4-6**

## WILD MUSHROOM-SPINACH LASAGNA

### AF (Dairy-free, Egg-free**, Corn-free, Gluten-free)

1 (10 ounce) package frozen chopped spinach, thawed and drained;
   or two bunches fresh spinach, cleaned, stems removed, and chopped
1 package of Rice lasagna noodles, cooked a la dente (do not use no-boil noodles)
½ cup Manchego cheese, grated (sheep)
3 cups Goat Gouda, shredded
3 cups milk substitute
2 tablespoons white rice flour
½ teaspoon salt
¼ teaspoon white pepper
1 tablespoon Pecorino Romano cheese, shredded
2 portabella mushrooms, stems removed, coarsely chopped
1 ounce dried wild mushrooms, rehydrated in hot water for 20 minutes,
   stems removed and chopped, reserve liquid
1 ounce dried porcini mushrooms, rehydrated in same hot water as above mushrooms
½ cup Madeira
¾ cube margarine, milk-free, corn-free
3 garlic cloves, minced
2 leeks, sliced vertically in half, then sliced (use only the white portion)
2/3 package of tofu, firm, drained
1 tablespoon miso
1 egg white
2 tablespoons parsley, chopped

**Cheeses:** In small separate bowl, mix Manchego and Gouda cheeses.
Spinach: Cook spinach according to package instructions. Drain and set aside. For fresh spinach see instructions following mushroom sauce.

**Mushroom sauce:** In large skillet, melt 4 tablespoons margarine. Add leeks and garlic, sauté until tender. Add mushrooms and cook until tender. Add Madeira and heat for 2 minutes. Remove mixture to separate bowl. If using fresh spinach, place prepared spinach in skillet that mushrooms were in, add a tablespoon of olive oil and cook until limp. Remove from skillet; set aside.

**Béchamel Sauce:** In that same skillet, melt remaining 2 tablespoons of margarine. Add flour and then slowly add milk substitute. Add salt, white pepper, and the Romano cheese; simmer, stirring constantly until slightly thickened. Remove from heat and set aside.

**Tofu mixture:** Into food processor add tofu, miso, parsley, and egg white. Pulse 30 seconds or until smooth. Remove and put into separate bowl.

**Assemble lasagna:** First place ½ cup of béchamel sauce on bottom of 13 by 9 baking dish. Then mix the cooked spinach into rest of béchamel sauce. Place 3 noodles on top of the sauce, next place ½ of the béchamel sauce, 1/2 of the tofu mixture, ½ of the mushroom sauce and 1/3 of Manchego and Gouda cheese mixture. Top with 3 more noodles. This time place rest of tofu mixture, followed by rest of mushroom sauce, and 1/3 of both cheeses. Add final layer of noodles, top with béchamel sauce and cheeses. Cover lasagna with foil. Bake in preheat oven of 375 degrees for 20 minutes. Remove foil and let bake another 15 to 20 minutes or until golden on top. Let sit 5-10 minutes before serving.
**Serves 8**

## STIR-FRIED VEGETABLES

### AF (Dairy-free, Egg-free, Corn-free, Gluten-free)

2 tablespoons tamari soy sauce (organic/wheat-free)
¼ cup dry sherry
¼ teaspoon salt
¼ teaspoon ginger, ground
¼ cup Beef stock* or Chicken stock* (or broth)
2 tablespoons canola oil or grape seed oil (good for cooking at high heat)
1 tablespoon sesame oil
2 garlic cloves, minced
6 cups assorted cut vegetables, washed and thoroughly dried, cut into small pieces for fast cooking
¼ cup almonds, sliced (optional)

Combine tamari, sherry, salt, ginger and stock or broth in small bowl. Set aside. Combine the two oils. Preheat a wok or large skillet to medium high heat. When hot add 1½ tablespoons oil and some of the minced garlic. The next part is quickly done, so all vegetables need to be prepared and ready. First add vegetables that take longer to cook, like carrots, green beans and broccoli. Turn and flip the vegetables in the hot oil. Then add green pepper, asparagus, celery, snow peas, and Chinese pea pods, continually to rapidly stir. Fast cooking vegetables like cabbage, mushrooms, green onions, bean sprouts and zucchini can be added toward the end of the cooking time. Tomatoes, water chestnuts, bamboo shoots need only to be warmed. Serve vegetables over rice.

**Serves 8**

## EGGPLANT PARMIGIANA

To make this recipe AF you will need mozzarella made from buffalo's milk. This cheese can be found at Italian delis. Also use egg whites instead of whole eggs.

### AF (Dairy-free (see note above), Egg-free**, Corn-free, Gluten-free)

1 pound eggplant, peeled and cut into ½ slices
3 egg whites beaten
2 cups rice bread crumbs or rice thins, finely ground
½ cup olive oil
½ cup Romano cheese (sheep), grated
1 teaspoon oregano
½ teaspoon garlic powder
2 tablespoons parsley, chopped
2 cups mozzarella cheese (only buffalo milk cheese from Italian delis)
1 (28 ounce) can tomato puree

Preheat oven to 350 degrees. Grease 8 by 8 baking dish. In separate bowl, mix oregano, garlic powder, and parsley, with grated Romano cheese. Place beaten egg whites in shallow dish. Place bread crumbs in separate shallow dish. Dip eggplant slices first into eggs, then into rice crumbs until coated. In large skillet, heat oil to medium high. Fry eggplant in hot oil until golden. Drain eggplant on paper towels. Arrange half of the eggplant slices in baking dish. Sprinkle 1/3 of cheese mixture on eggplant slices and ¼ cup of mozzarella cheese. Special note: this cheese has a great deal of liquid to it. Use your hands to break it up. Next pour ½ of tomato puree over slices. Repeat procedure for next layer. Top with last 1/3 of cheese mixture. Bake uncovered for 25 minutes. Top with last ¼ cup of mozzarella cheese and cook another 5 minutes or until cheese is melted.

**Serves 8**

## WILD MUSHROOMS AND POLENTA

**T (Testing for corn—Dairy-free, Egg-free, Gluten-free)**

**Mushroom mixture:**

2 tablespoons margarine, milk-free

2 portabella mushrooms, stems removed, coarsely chopped

1 ounce package dried porcini mushrooms, soaking in hot water 20 minutes

1 cup onion, chopped

½ cup Madeira

¼ cup beef broth, have more on hand if necessary

3 fresh garlic cloves, pressed

½ teaspoon thyme

¼ teaspoon salt

¼ teaspoon pepper

1 bay leaf

In medium size skillet, melt margarine. Place onions in pan and sauté until tender. Remove stems of porcini mushrooms and chop. Add porcini and portabella mushrooms and cook until tender about 2 minutes adding more margarine if necessary. Add garlic and sauté 30 seconds, add Madeira, beef broth, spices, bay leaf, salt and pepper and simmer for 10 minutes. Remove bay leaf. Meanwhile, prepare polenta.

**Polenta:**

One precooked polenta tube

2 tablespoons grape seed oil or canola oil

Slice cooked polenta into ½ inches. Lay on paper towels for ½ hour. Press paper towels on polenta to remove excess liquid. Place oil in 12 inch skillet and heat to medium-high. Pan Fry polenta slices until heated thoroughly, approximately 5 minutes on each side.

**To Serve:**

Spoon Mushroom sauce over polenta. Serve warm.

**Serves 6**

## PORTABELLA MUSHROOM AND ROASTED PEPPER SANDWICH

### AF (Dairy-free, Egg-free, Corn-free, Gluten-free)

4 portabella mushrooms, sliced
1 (15 ounce) jar of roasted red peppers
1 (4 ounce) Gouda goat cheese, sliced
3 sprigs of fresh rosemary
1 garlic clove, minced
½ to ¾ cup olive oil
8 slices of commercial rice bread (Ener-g rice bread is the best,
  do not use frozen is possible)
½ cup eggless mayonnaise (Vegenaise is a good choice) optional
2 to 3 tablespoons commercial pesto (read label) optional see note*
½ teaspoon sugar (optional)

In small bowl, mix mayonnaise and sugar with pesto. Set aside. In small sauce pan, add olive oil, salt and pepper and rosemary sprigs. Heat mixture for 20 minutes. Meanwhile in small skillet with small amount of oil, sauté Portabella mushrooms with the garlic. Set aside. Place rice bread on cookie sheets and brush with oil cooked with rosemary. Brush both side of bread, place in preheat oven of 375 degrees and bake 7–10 minutes on each side. Meanwhile, in small skillet with 1 tablespoon oil, sauté garlic and mushrooms until tender. Keep warm. Remove roasted pepper from jar, place in microwave dish and microwave 30 second to 1 minute on HIGH or until warm. Remove rice bread from oven, assemble sandwich the following method. First, spread mayonnaise, pesto mixture on cooked rice bread, then place portabella mushroom, slice of goat cheese, and warm roasted red peppers. This is also good without the pesto-mayonnaise dressing.

**Makes 4 sandwiches**

Note:* Most commercial pesto contains vinegar to help keep the pesto fresh.
I add the sugar to offset the vinegar.

123

## ZUCCHINI BOATS

### AF (Dairy-free, Egg-free, Corn-free, Gluten-free)

4 medium zucchinis
$\frac{1}{4}$ cup margarine, milk-free, corn-free
$\frac{1}{4}$ cup green onions, chopped
$\frac{1}{2}$ pound fresh mushroom, sliced
1 cup almonds, chopped
$\frac{1}{2}$ cup cooked rice
2 tablespoons parsley, chopped
1 tablespoon paprika
1 tablespoon tamari soy sauce (organic/wheat-free)

Cut zucchinis in half lengthwise. Boil zucchinis until tender; drain and cool. Scoop out cooked zucchini mulch and mash, reserving the shells. Melt margarine in a skillet and sauté onions, and mushroom until tender. In a mixing bowl, mix mashed zucchini with mushrooms and onion. Add almonds, cooked rice, parsley, and tamari. Place zucchini boats in a low pan, and fill each boat with some zucchini mixture. Sprinkle tops with paprika. Bake 20 minutes at 350 degrees.
**Serves 6**

## PORTABELLA MUSHROOM AND ARTICHOKE PIZZA

**(Corn-free, Gluten-free)**

**Pizza Dough:**
Look for a package of Gluten-free pizza mix and follow instructions (most gluten-free mix may have milk and egg products in it)

**Sauce:**
In a sauce pan, combine 2 cups tomato sauce, t teaspoon oregano, 1 teaspoon Italian seasoning, ¼ cup water, 1 teaspoon thyme, ½ teaspoon garlic salt and pepper. Bring mixture to boiling. Reduce heat to simmer and allow to thicken.

**Topping:**
2 green pepper, sliced (precook in microwave for 30 seconds)
1 (4.5 ounce) can black olives, sliced
½ pound portabella mushrooms, stem removed, sliced
½ onion, sliced
2 cups Mozzarella cheese
½ cup grated Romano cheese
1 jar marinated artichokes, drained, sliced

Prepare pizza dough as instructed on pizza package. Spread out on a pizza pan or cookie sheet. Pour sauce on top. Top with Mozzarella cheese, mushrooms, green peppers, artichokes and olives. Finish with grated Romano cheese. Bake at temperature suggest by pizza package.
**Serves 4-6**

## RICE PIE

**T (Testing for eggs—Dairy-free, Corn-free, Gluten-free)**

3 tablespoons olive oil
2 cups cooked rice
2 medium zucchinis, sliced and then halved
½ cup carrots, grated
1 garlic clove, minced
½ cup green onion, chopped
¼ cup parsley, chopped
6 eggs, beaten
1 teaspoon oregano
½ teaspoon thyme
1 teaspoon salt
½ teaspoon pepper
½ cup rice thins, ground
2 cup Manchego cheese, grated (sheep)
1 tablespoon margarine, milk-free, corn-free, melted

Preheat oven to 350 degrees. In large skillet, add oil and sauté onions, and garlic. Add zucchinis and carrots and cook until tender. In large mixing bowl, beat eggs, add cooked rice (cooled), and cheese. Add sautéed vegetable mixture to egg/rice mixture. In greased glass pie dish, pour mixture into pie dish. Sprinkle rice thins on top. Place melted margarine over the rice mixture. Bake at 350 degree for 40 to 50 minutes.

**Serves 6**

## VEGETARIAN STEW

### AF (Dairy-free, Egg-free, Corn-free, Gluten-free)

2 tablespoons margarine, milk-free, corn-free
1 red onion, chopped
1 teaspoon thyme
Bouquet Garni*
4 cups tomato juice
1 turnip, peeled, chopped
1 cup celery, sliced
1 pound red potatoes, peeled and cut into chunks
6 carrots, peeled, cut in half and then julienned
1 (15 ounce) can garbanzo beans
1 cup rice thins, ground
2 tablespoons parsley, chopped
½ cup Manchego cheese, (imported/sheep)

In a Dutch oven, melt margarine: add onion and sauté. Add thyme, bouquet gar-ni*, tomato juice, turnip, celery, potatoes, and carrots. Bring to broil. Cover, reduce heat and simmer 30 minutes or until potatoes and carrots are just tender. Uncover and add garbanzo beans. Cook and reduce liquid. Top with ground rice thins, mixed with cheese, and sprinkle with parsley.
**Serves 6**

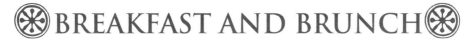

# ✳BREAKFAST AND BRUNCH✳

## BREAKFAST BREAD PUDDING

### AF (Dairy-free, Egg-free**, Corn-free, Gluten-free)

2 egg whites
2 cups milk substitute, vanilla soy milk works well
½ cup brown sugar
1 teaspoon cinnamon
¼ teaspoon nutmeg
4 cups dry rice bread cubes
¼ cup raisins, currants or chopped dates
¼ cup almonds, chopped

Beat egg whites in mixing bowl; add milk substitute, brown sugar and spices. Place bread cubes in a greased 9 by 13 baking dish. Pour mixture over bread cubes. Cover and let stand at least 30 minutes. Remove cover. Top with fruit and almonds. Place in a pre-heated oven of 350 degrees. Bake for 20 minutes.
**Serves 4**

## BLUEBBERRY RICE PUDDING

### AF (Dairy-free, Egg-free**, Corn-free, Gluten-free)

2 cups cooked rice, short grained like rose, no processed rice
2 cups milk substitute, vanilla soy works the best
Dash of salt
½ cup sugar
2 egg whites, beaten
1/8 teaspoon lemon zest
½ cup frozen blueberries, thawed
¼ cup almonds, finely chopped

In large mixing bowl, mix rice, milk substitute, salt, sugar, egg whites, and zest. In greased 1½ quart casserole dish place one half of the mixture, layer ¼ cup of blueberries on top of rice mixture. Repeat layers and top with chopped almonds. Bake in preheated oven of 350 degrees, for 20 minutes.
**Serves 4**

## CINNAMON AND FRUIT OATMEAL

### AF (Dairy-free, Egg-free, Corn-free, Gluten-free)

1 cup rolled oatmeal, organic, not instant
1 ¾ cup milk substitute or water
½ teaspoon cinnamon
¼ teaspoon nutmeg
¼ cup brown sugar
Dash of salt
¼ to ½ cup of fresh or thawed frozen berries (blueberry, raspberry, etc)

In medium saucepan, bring liquid (water or milk substitute) to boil. Dissolve sugar in liquid. Add oats, salt and spices, and stir for 1 to 2 minutes. Add fruit and allow to heat. Serve hot. **Serves 2-3**

## LOX AND RICE BREAD

To make this AF, goat cheese is needed until corn is tested. Then you can use tofutti cream cheese instead.

### AF (Dairy-free, Egg-free**, Corn-free, Gluten-free)

4 slices of rice bread, toasted
½ cup goat cheese, Gouda is nice, later on use cream cheese substitute
3 ounces sliced smoked salmon
¼ of red onion, sliced and cooked in microwave 15 second

Place toasted bread on plates. Spread goat cheese on each piece. Follow with slice of salmon and red onion.
**Serves 4**

**RICEOLA CEREAL**

**AF (Dairy-free, Egg-free, Corn-free, Gluten-free)**

2 cups puffed brown rice
2 cups puffed millet
½ cup sliced almonds
¼ cup sesame seeds
¼ cup brown sugar
¼ cup dried fruit, raisins, apricots, dried cherries, dried cranberries, etc.

In large bowl, mix all ingredients together. Serve with milk substitute.
**Serves 6**

**APPLE CRISP**
This is either dessert or breakfast item. It is also listed in the dessert section.

**AF (Dairy-free, Egg-free, Corn-free, Gluten-free)**

4 apples, cored, peeled, and sliced
2 tablespoons margarine, milk-free, corn-free
1 teaspoon cinnamon
Dash salt
½ cup brown sugar
1 cup oats, rolled and uncooked
1 tablespoon sorghum flour
1 teaspoon lemon juice

Place sliced apples in greased 8 by 8 inch baking dish. Sprinkle with lemon juice. Mix the rest of the ingredients in small mixing bowl and sprinkle over apples. Bake in pre-heated oven of 350 degree for 20 minutes or until just golden brown.
**Variations:** To use fresh peaches or cherries, increase the brown sugar to ¾ cup.
**Serves 6**

**ALLOWED CEREALS**

**AF (Dairy-free, Egg-free, Corn-free, Gluten-free)**

1. Buckwheat (kasha)
2. Puffed rice
3. Puffed millet

**DAY BEFORE JALAPENO EGG CASSEROLE**

**T (Testing for egg—Dairy-free, Corn-free, Gluten-free)**

1 cube margarine, softened, milk-free, corn-free
7 slices of commercial rice bread, not frozen (Ener-g is the best so far)
2 ½ cups of goat Jalapeno cheese, shredded
10 eggs
2 cups non-dairy milk (soy works best)
2 teaspoons ground chipotle chili pepper
¼ teaspoon cumin
½ cup onion, finely chopped
1 teaspoon salt
¼ teaspoon pepper

Grease 9 by 13 inch baking pan. In bowl, mix egg together with whisk. Next add non-dairy milk, chipotle pepper, cumin, onion, salt and pepper to eggs. Meanwhile, spread margarine over slices of rice bread. Cut bread into cubes. Place ½ of the bread cubes into baking pan. Sprinkle ½ of the cheese over the bread. Repeat the process with the remaining bread and cheese. Pour egg mixture over cheese and bread cubes. Cover tightly and put in refrigerator until the next day. Give it at least 24 hours to soak. To bake, preheat oven to 350 degrees. Bake for 45 minutes to 1 hour, or until golden brown and consistency is firm. Serve warm.
**Serve 8**

## ORANGE FRENCH TOAST

**T (Testing for eggs—Dairy-free, Corn-free, Gluten-free)**

8 slices Gluten-free bread, sliced into ½ inch
6 eggs, beaten
¾ cup milk substitute, vanilla soy milk is good
¼ cup orange juice
½ teaspoon vanilla
2 tablespoons margarine, milk-free, corn-free
  Maple syrup
  Powdered sugar

In large bowl, mix eggs, milk substitute, orange juice and vanilla. Place slices of bread into 2 baking dishes. Pour mixture over bread slices. Allow to soak for 30 minutes for homemade bread and 2 to 4 hours for commercial bread (my husband thinks the homemade bread makes better toast). On hot large skillet or stove griddle, melt margarine. Place bread slices and cook for 4 minutes on each side. Work in batches and repeat procedure with second batch. Warm in oven the first batch of French toast. Serve hot. Top slices with either maple syrup or powdered sugar.
**Serves 4**

## CRUMB TOPPING COFFEE CAKE

**AF (Dairy-free, Egg-free\*\*, Corn-free, Gluten-free)**

2/3 cup white rice flour
½ cup brown rice flour
1/3 cup sorghum flour          **} or 1 3/4 cup of Terry's Flour Blend**
2 tablespoons potato starch
2 tablespoons tapioca flour
1 teaspoon xanthan gum
1 ½ teaspoon baking powder
¼ teaspoon salt
½ teaspoon cinnamon
¼ teaspoon nutmeg (optional)
2 egg whites, beaten
2/3 cup sugar
4 tablespoons margarine, milk-free, corn-free
1 to 1/3 cup milk substitute

In large mixing bowl, mix 5 first ingredients together. Remove ¼ cup of mixture and put in small mixing bowl for crumb topping. Set aside. To remaining mixture, add the xanthan gum, baking powder, salt, cinnamon, and nutmeg. Mix and put mixture on large sheet of wax paper. In another large mixing bowl, cream margarine and sugar together until smooth. Add egg and mix together. Add flour mixture and milk substitute into sugar mixture 1/3 at a time. Place in greased 9 by 9 by 2 inch baking pan. Top with Crumb Topping*. Place in preheated oven of 350 degrees and bake 30 to 35 minutes. Cool and serve.

**Crumb Topping**
¼ cup reserved flour mix
2 tablespoons margarine, softened, cut into small dots
3 tablespoon brown sugar
½ teaspoon cinnamon

In small bowl that reserved ¼ cup of mixed flour was already in, add brown sugar, and cinnamon. Mix ingredients until crumbly. Sprinkle topping on coffee cake batter. Dot topping with margarine. Bake in preheated oven of 350 degrees for 30 to 35 minutes.

## SHREDDED APPLE MUFFINS

### AF (Dairy-free, Egg-free**, Corn-free, Gluten-free)

2/3 cup white rice flour
½ cup brown rice flour
1/3 cup sorghum flour          } **or 1 3/4 cup of Terry's Flour Blend**
2 tablespoons potato starch
2 tablespoons tapioca flour
1 teaspoon xanthan gum
1 teaspoon baking powder
1 teaspoon baking soda
1 teaspoon cinnamon
½ teaspoon nutmeg
½ teaspoon salt
2 egg whites, beaten
¾ cup sugar
1/3 cup canola oil
1 teaspoon vanilla
½ cup milk substitute
2/3 cup shredded apples

In separate bowl, measure and mix top 5 flours together. Remove ¼ cup of mixed flours and set aside. Add to remaining flours xanthan gum, baking powder, baking soda, spices, and salt. Set aside.

In another bowl, beat oil, vanilla, and sugar until thick and creamy. Add beaten egg whites. Beat in milk.

**Grate apple.** Set aside. Add the egg mixture to the flour mixture one third at a time. Mix thoroughly. Mix in the shredded apple. Add the extra flour only if batter seems too thin. Pour batter into greased muffin tins and bake in preheated oven of 350 degrees for 15 to 20 minutes. Remove from oven when a wooden toothpick comes out clean.

**Makes 12 muffins**

## APRICOT NUT BREAD

**AF (Dairy-free, Egg-free**, Corn-free, Gluten-free)**

2/3 cup sweet rice flour
½ cup brown rice flour
1/3 cup sorghum
2 tablespoons potato starch
2 tablespoons tapioca flour

**or 1 3/4 cup of Terry's Flour Blend**

1 teaspoon xanthan gum
1 ½ teaspoon baking powder
1 teaspoon baking soda
½ teaspoon salt
½ teaspoon cinnamon
1/3 cup apricots, chopped and dried
2 tablespoon raisins
2 to 3 egg whites
½ cup sugar
1/3 cup vegetable oil
1 teaspoon vanilla
½ cup to 1 cup milk substitute
¼ cup chopped almonds

On wax paper, mix flours together: brown rice, sweet rice, potato starch and tapioca flour. Remove from mixture ¼ cup and set aside. To remaining flour mixture, add : xanthan gum, baking powder, soda, spices and salt to flour mixture on wax paper. In large mixing bowl, mix eggs whites, oil and vanilla. Add sugar to mix and beat until creamy. Add milk substitute. Add flour mixture to egg mixture alittle at a time while beating with mixer. If too runny add reserve flour mixture. If mixture looks good do not add remaining flour. Bake in a greased dark loaf pan, at 350 degrees for 40 minutes.
**Makes 1 loaf**

# PASTA, RICE & GRAIN DISHES

## PASTA DISHES

The new brown rice pasta makes a very enjoyable pasta. The rice pasta is made from either Organic Brown rice or Stone—ground rice pasta. Either one is delicious, though it takes about 10 minutes longer to cook.

**PENNE PASTA WITH CHICKEN AND LEEKS**

**AF (Dairy-free, Egg-free, Corn-free, Gluten-free)**
2 tablespoons oil
4 boneless chicken breasts, skinless
   salt and pepper
4 tablespoons margarine, milk-free, corn-free
2 cups leeks, chopped, white area only
4 garlic cloves, minced
1 twenty-eight ounce can tomatoes, drained or 4 tomatoes, quartered
¼ cup dry vermouth
1 pound rice penne pasta
¾ cup Romano cheese, grated

In large skillet, heat oil. Salt and pepper the chicken. Add prepared chicken and cook leeks on both sides until brown. Remove from skillet and set aside. Slice or quarter chicken. Add more olive oil to skillet. Cook in chicken dripping until tender, about 7 to 10 minutes. Add tomatoes, vermouth, and chicken. Heat chicken mixture for 15 minutes. Toss chicken mixture with cooked penne. Serve and top with Romano.
**Serves 4**

## TURKEY SAUSAGE MILANO

### AF (Dairy-free, Egg-free, Corn-free, Gluten-free)

3 to 4 links of Italian turkey sausage, skin removed and crumbled
1/3 cup olive oil
1 cup green pepper, chopped
1 ½ cup green onion, chopped
½ cup parsley, chopped
1 eight ounce can tomato sauce
3 garlic cloves, minced
1 teaspoon dried basil
1 teaspoon dried oregano
½ teaspoon rosemary
1 pound rice pasta, any variety
  freshly grated Romano cheese

In large skillet, cook turkey sausage until brown. Remove sausage with slotted spoon (there will not be a great deal of grease). Drain on paper towels. Add margarine and melt in skillet. Add green onions and green peppers. Sauté onions and peppers until tender. Add tomato sauce, salt and pepper, and rest of spices. Add sausage back into mixture. Cover and simmer mixture for 30 minutes.

Meanwhile cook pasta in large quart pan in boiling water (remember this pasta takes longer to cook than regular pasta). Serve mixture over rice pasta.
**Serves 6**

## CHICKEN PASTA W/GOAT CHEESE

### AF (Dairy-free, Egg-free, Corn-free, Gluten-free)

4 tablespoons olive oil
4 tablespoons margarine, milk-free, corn-free
5 ounces creamy goat cheese
1 cup toasted (gluten-free) breadcrumbs, or rice thins, ground
1 red bell pepper, sliced
2 onions, diced
4 chicken breasts, skinless, sliced
12 ounces rice pasta, spirals
**Dressing:**
½ cup balsamic vinegar
¼ cup olive oil

In separate bowl, mix vinegar and olive oil. Mix well. Set aside. Heat olive oil and margarine in skillet over medium heat. Add red pepper and onion, cook for about 10 minutes, stirring occasionally. Remove vegetables with slotted spoon and set aside. Raise heat on skillet to medium- high; add chicken and sauté on both sides until done. Meanwhile cook rice pasta for 20 minutes or until done. Mix pasta, vegetables, chicken, and then toss with the goat cheese mixture and dressing.
**Serves 4**

## MACARONI AND CHEESE WITH LEEKS

My husband especially loves the taste with the leeks and goat cheese.

### AF (Dairy-free, Egg-free, Corn-free, Gluten-free)

2/3 cup leeks, sliced vertically, sliced and chopped
3 tablespoons margarine, milk-free, corn-free
3 tablespoons white rice flour
1 cup milk substitute, soy, almond or rice
½ teaspoon salt
¼ teaspoon pepper
½ cup dry white wine
1 cup goat cheddar cheese, grated*
2/3 cup goat jack cheese, grated
1 ½ cups rice macaroni pasta, cooked al dente about 12 to 17 minutes

Melt margarine in large skillet. Add leeks and sauté until tender. Add rice flour
to leeks. Slowly add milk substitute to avoid lumps. Add wine, salt and pepper.
Cook over medium-high heat stirring constantly until thickened. Add cheeses and
stir until melted. Place cooked macaroni in 1¾ quart greased casserole dish. Add
cheese mixture and stir into macaroni. Place casserole dish in preheated oven of
350 degrees. Baked uncovered for about 35 minutes.

**Serves 4**

*Goat cheese can be salty, you may want to lessen the amount of salt to ¼ teaspoon.

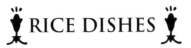

# RICE DISHES

## BASIC STOVE TOP RICE

### AF (Dairy-free, Egg-free, Corn-free, Gluten-free)

1 cup rice
2 cups boiling water
2 tablespoon margarine, milk-free, corn-free
½ teaspoon salt

Bring water margarine, and salt to boil. Add rice stir once, lower heat and cook covered for 20 minutes. Do not look at the rice while it is cooking. Remove from heat and allow to steam for 5 minutes.
**Makes 3 cups**

## BASIC BASMATI RICE

### AF (Dairy-free, Egg-free, Corn-free, Gluten-free)

2 tablespoons margarine, milk-free, corn-free (optional)
1 cup Basmati rice (either white or brown)
2 cups water or broth

In 1 to 2 quart sauce pan, combine rice and water. Bring to boil. Reduce to simmer. Cover and cook for 50 minutes. Remove from heat. Let stand for 5 to 10 minutes.
**Serves 4-6**

## CHINESE FRIED RICE

### (Dairy-free, Corn-free, Gluten-free)

5 tablespoons margarine, milk-free, corn-free
½ cup shallots, chopped
½ cup almonds, sliced
½ cup celery, sliced
½ cup green pepper, finely chopped
½ cup mushrooms, sliced
2 eggs, slightly beaten
3 cups cooked rice
2 tablespoons tamari soy sauce (traditional/wheat-free)

In large skillet, melt 2 tablespoons margarine. Add shallots, green pepper and celery, and mushrooms, sauté until tender. Remove from skillet and set aside. Add 2 additional tablespoons of margarine to skillet, add eggs, and stir slightly until set. Remove eggs from skillet and slice into strips. Add remaining tablespoon of margarine, add rice and stir-fry rice until well heated. Add vegetable mixture and sliced eggs back to skillet. Stir in tamari. Stir-fry 1 to 2 minutes until heated thoroughly.
**Serves 4**

## CURRIED RICE

### AF (Dairy-free, Egg-free, Corn-free, Gluten-free)

2 tablespoons margarine, milk-free, corn-free
¼ cup onion, chopped
1 teaspoon curry powder
½ teaspoon salt
¼ teaspoon pepper
3 cups cooked rice
½ cup almonds, sliced

In a large skillet, melt margarine. Add onion and curry and sauté until tender. Add rice, salt and pepper and stir. Cook until thoroughly heated. Sprinkle almonds over rice mixture. Serve hot.
**Serves 4**

## SPANISH RICE

**AF (Dairy-free, Egg-free, Corn-free, Gluten-free)**

2 tablespoons margarine, milk-free, corn-free
1 cup uncooked rice
8 ounces tomato sauce
½ teaspoon chili powder
½ teaspoon salt
1 cup water

Melt margarine in large skillet, and brown rice. Add tomato sauce, water, chili powder, and salt, bring to boil. Reduce heat, cover and simmer for 20 minutes.
**Serves 4**

## ALMONDS AND WILD RICE

**AF (Dairy-free, Egg-free, Corn-free, Gluten-free)**

1 cup wild rice, rinsed twice
4 tablespoons margarine, milk-free, corn-free
½ cup celery, chopped
½ cup almonds, sliced
½ cup mushrooms, sliced
¼ cup shallots, chopped
2 cups Chicken Stock* or chicken broth

In large skillet, add 2 tablespoon margarine. Sauté wild rice in margarine until lightly brown. Push rice to the side or remove and set aside. Add 2 more tablespoons margarine and sauté, shallots, celery, mushrooms until tender. Add chicken stock or broth, cover and simmer 30 to 40 minutes or until rice is fluffy.
**Serves 4**

## MANCHEGO RISOTTO

### AF (Dairy-free, Egg-free, Corn-free, Gluten-free)

1 cup Arborio rice, uncooked
2 tablespoon margarine, melted, milk-free, corn-free
1 tablespoon olive oil
¾ cup onion, chopped
1 clove garlic, minced
3 cups chicken or beef broth, heated
¼ teaspoon salt
2 tablespoons freshly grated Manchego cheese, sheep

Melt margarine in large skillet, add oil, and then add rice. Cook rice in margarine-oil mixture stirring constantly until the rice is white (you really need to watch someone do this to understand the color of the rice). Add onion and garlic and sauté until tender. Add broth one cup at a time, stirring constantly until the broth is absorbed. This process takes about 30 to 40 minutes. Remove from heat. Stir in salt and cheese.
**Serves 6**

For a variation add Portobello mushroom. In separate skillet add olive oil, place chopped mushroom in skillet and sauté. Add chopped mushroom after salt and cheese.

# ❧ GRAIN DISHES ❧

## POLENTA

With the new instant polentas, this grain if easy to fix.

### T (Testing for corn—Dairy-free, Egg-free, Gluten-free)

1 cup Instant Polenta
1 quart water
1 teaspoon salt

In large sauce pan, bring water to boil. Slowly add polenta stirring constantly. Instant take about 3 minutes to thicken. Stir until consistency desired.
**Serves 6**

## FRIED POLENTA

### T (Testing for corn—Dairy-free, Egg-free, Gluten-free)

Cooled polenta, cut into ½ inch slices
½ to 1 cup olive oil

In large skillet, heat oil until hot. Place slices of polenta into oil, cook until a slight crust forms, then turn over and do other side. Transfer to paper towels to drain.
**Serves 4-6**

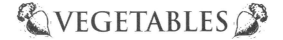

# VEGETABLES

## LIMA BEANS WITH TURKEY BACON

### AF (Dairy-free, Egg-free, Corn-free, Gluten-free)

1 (10 ounce) package of frozen lima beans
4 slices of turkey bacon, thinly sliced
2 tablespoon olive oil
¼ cup shallots, chopped
1 garlic clove, minced
½ teaspoon salt
¼ teaspoon pepper

Prepare lima beans according to package instructions. Set aside. In large skillet, cook bacon until done, remove with slotted spoon. Add olive oil to pan, sauté shallots and garlic until tender. Add lima beans to skillet with salt and pepper. Cook until heated. Serve with bacon sprinkled on top.
**Serves 4**

## CROOK-NECK SQUASH WITH RED ONIONS

### AF (Dairy-free, Egg-free, Corn-free, Gluten-free)

3 crook-neck squash, sliced
¼ cup margarine, milk-free, corn-free
2 garlic cloves, minced
1 cup red onion, finely chopped
2 tablespoons parsley, chopped

In large skillet, melt margarine. Add red onion and sauté until tender. Add sliced squash and garlic and cook until squash is soft and tender. Top with parsley.
**Serves 4**

## GREEN BEAN ALMONDINE

### AF (Dairy-free, Egg-free, Corn-free, Gluten-free)

1 ½ pounds green beans, tips broken off
3 tablespoons margarine, milk-free, corn-free
1 cup fresh mushrooms, sliced
½ cup almonds, sliced
1 garlic clove, minced
¼ teaspoon salt
¼ teaspoon pepper

Steam green beans until tender. Remove from steamer. In large skillet, melt margarine and sauté mushrooms and garlic for 1 to 2 minutes. Add green beans, salt and pepper. Cook until thoroughly heated.
**Serves 6**

## GINGER GLAZED CARROTS

### AF (Dairy-free, Egg-free, Corn-free, Gluten-free)

4 tablespoon margarine, milk-free, corn-free, or oil
¼ cup red onion, chopped
2 tablespoon brown sugar
¼ cup orange juice
1 tablespoon fresh ginger, grated
2 pound carrots, peeled, sliced

Steam carrots until tender. In large skillet melt margarine, add red onion and sauté until tender. Add orange juice, ginger, and brown sugar. Stir until sugars are dissolved. Add cooked carrots and toss until coated with glaze. Serve warm.
**Serves 6**

## CARROT AND CAULIFOWER ROMANO

### AF (Dairy-free, Egg-free, Corn-free, Gluten-free)

6 fresh carrots, cut into strips
1 head of cauliflower
2 to 3 tablespoons margarine, milk-free, corn-free
2 garlic cloves, minced
2 tablespoons parsley, chopped
3 tablespoons freshly grated Romano cheese (imported/sheep)

Wash, peel, and cut carrots into 2-inch long strips. Wash cauliflower and separate into flowerets. Place carrots in steamer, cover and cook 5 minutes, then add the cauliflower and cook an addition 5 minutes or until both carrots and cauliflower are just done. Do not overcook.

In skillet, melt margarine and sauté cooked carrots and cauliflower with garlic over low heat. Remove mixture to a serving dish, top with parsley and Romano cheese.
**Serves 6**

## STEWED EGGPLANT

### AF (Dairy-free, Egg-free, Corn-free, Gluten-free)

2 tablespoons margarine, milk-free, corn-free
½ cup onion, chopped
1 large eggplant, peeled and cut into 1-inch cubes
1 teaspoon salt
¼ teaspoon pepper
½ cup water
2 tablespoons lemon juice
1/8 teaspoon allspice

In 10-inch skillet, melt margarine. Add onion and sauté until tender. Add eggplant, salt, pepper, water, lemon juice, and allspice. Simmer until tender.
**Serves 6**

## ARTICHOKES WITH LIMA BEANS

### AF (Dairy-free, Egg-free, Corn-free, Gluten-free)

1 (10 ounce) package frozen artichoke hearts
1 (10 ounce) package lima beans
3 tablespoons margarine, milk-free, corn-free
$\frac{1}{2}$ cup green onions, chopped
1 garlic clove, minced
1 cup carrot, diced
1 cup celery, diced
$\frac{1}{2}$ cup tomato sauce
$\frac{1}{2}$ teaspoon salt
$\frac{1}{4}$ teaspoon thyme
Water

Thaw artichokes and lima beans. In a large skillet, melt margarine. Add carrots first and sauté for 5 minutes, then add onions, garlic, and celery. Sauté mixture until the vegetables are tender. Add tomato sauce, salt, and thyme. Add artichokes, lima beans, and enough water just to cover artichokes. Cover and simmer for 20 minutes or until artichokes and lima beans are tender.
**Serves 6-8**

## SKILLET RED POTATOES

### AF (Dairy-free, Egg-free, Corn-free, Gluten-free)

1 ½ to 2 pounds red potatoes, cut into 1-inch wedges (Do not peel!)
2 tablespoons olive oil
1 garlic clove, minced
1 teaspoon thyme, dried
¼ teaspoon paprika
¼ teaspoon salt
1/8 teaspoon pepper

In microwavable bowl, mix potatoes with olive oil, salt and pepper. Cover with plastic wrap. Microwave potatoes 10 to 12 minutes on high. At 5 minutes, take the bowl out and stir the potatoes. Put more plastic wrap on bowl, continue microwaving. Put another 2 tablespoons olive oil in 12-inch skillet. Add potatoes, garlic, thyme and paprika, and cook until golden about 10 minutes.

**Serves 6**

## POTATO BOATS

### (Egg-free, Corn-free, Gluten-free)

6 medium baking potatoes
¼ cup butter or margarine
½ cup green onions, sliced
1 teaspoon salt
¼ teaspoon pepper
½ cup milk
Dash paprika

Wash and dry potatoes: prick skins with a fork: bake about one hour at 425 degrees or until tender when pierced (Note: at trick when time is short, heat in microwave first and cook last half hour in oven). Allow potato to cool enough to handle. Cut lengthwise, divide each potato in half. With a spoon, scoop out halves to form 12 shells.

Melt margarine in small skillet. Add green onions and sauté until tender.

In large bowl, with mixer at low speed, beat potatoes, butter (or margarine) and onion mixture, salt, pepper and ¼ cup milk until smooth. Continue adding milk as needed. Spoon the mixture back into potato shells, and sprinkle a dash of paprika. Place on microwave-safe plate, and microwave at HIGH for one minute or until potatoes are thoroughly heated.
**Serves 12**

### Variations:
1. Cook sliced turkey bacon in skillet. Crumble turkey on top of prepared potato boats.
2. Add 1 cup canned salmon or fresh salmon, chopped, to mixture.
3. Add grated Romano or Manchego cheese to mixture.

## POTATO PANCAKES

### (Dairy-free, Corn -free, Gluten-free)

4 medium potatoes
2 tablespoons onion, grated
1 teaspoon salt
¼ teaspoon white pepper
1 tablespoon sorghum flour
2 eggs, well beaten
5 tablespoon oil (grape seed oil does well with high heat)

Peel potatoes and soak 1 hour. Grate potatoes, and press them in cheesecloth until all liquid is drained. Add onion, salt, white pepper, and flour. Mix well. Drop by spoonfuls onto a hot skillet with oil. Fry on both sides until golden.
**Serves 4**

## POTATOES WITH PARSLEY SAUCE

### AF (Dairy-free, Egg-free, Corn-free, Gluten-free)

4 tablespoon olive oil
5 boiling potatoes, peeled and sliced
1 garlic clove, minced
¼ cup fresh parsley, chopped
¼ cup pine nuts
1 teaspoon salt
1/8 teaspoon pepper
1 ¼ cup Chicken Stock* or chicken broth, hot

In large skillet, heat olive oil. Add potatoes, and cook over medium heat until they are golden brown. Push potatoes over to the side. Add garlic and onion and sauté until tender. Drain any excess oil. Add parsley, pine nuts, salt and pepper. Pour in hot chicken stock. Cover skillet and simmer over low heat for 25 minutes or until potatoes are tender. Transfer potato to a platter; pour the cooking liquid over them.
**Serves 4**

## FRESH SPINACH WITH ALMONDS AND PINE NUTS

### AF (Dairy-free, Egg-free, Corn-free, Gluten-free)

3 tablespoons olive oil
1 garlic clove, minced
¼ cup pine nuts
¼ cup almonds, sliced
1 pound fresh spinach, cleaned and stems removed
1 teaspoon salt

In large skillet, heat oil and sauté garlic for 1 minute. Add spinach, cook until limp. Add pine nuts and almonds to spinach and mix until heated.
**Serves 4**


## BAKED SQUASH

### AF (Dairy-free, Egg-free, Corn-free, Gluten-free)

1 medium acorn, sultan, yellow, summer or spaghetti squash
3 tablespoons margarine, milk-free, corn-free
   Salt and Pepper to taste

Preheat oven to 350 degrees. Prepare squash; cut into halves or quarters, and re-move seeds. Place squash skin down on greased baking dish. Bake for 30 minutes until tender. Dot with butter and serve.
**Serves 4**

## BAKED STUFFED TOMATOES

**AF (Dairy-free, Egg-free, Corn-free, Gluten-free)**

8 large tomatoes, cut in half
2 tablespoons margarine, milk-free, corn-free
$\frac{1}{2}$ cup shallots, finely chopped
2 garlic cloves, minced
$\frac{1}{4}$ cup parsley, chopped
$\frac{1}{2}$ teaspoon dried thyme
1/8 teaspoon oregano
$\frac{1}{2}$ cup rice thins, crumbled
$\frac{1}{2}$ teaspoon salt
$\frac{1}{4}$ teaspoon pepper
$\frac{1}{2}$ cup pine nuts

Wash tomatoes and cut them in half. Scoop out centers and place in a medium-size mixing bowl. In a small skillet, melt margarine, and sauté shallots and garlic until tender. Add shallots and garlic to mixing bowl. Then add parsley, thyme, oregano, rice thins, salt, pepper, and pine nuts. Mix ingredients well. Spoon some mixture into each tomato half. Place each stuffed tomato in a lightly greased baking dish or pan. Bake tomatoes at 425 degrees for 8 to 10 minutes or until tomatoes are softened.
**Serves 8**

## RATATOUILLE

### AF (Dairy-free, Egg-free, Corn-free, Gluten-free)

4 medium tomatoes
1 medium eggplant
4 tablespoons olive oil
1 large onion, sliced
2 zucchini, sliced
1 large green pepper, cut into strips
1 large red pepper, cut into strips
1 teaspoon dried basil
1 teaspoon Italian seasoning
1 teaspoon salt
Freshly ground pepper
½ cup white wine
2 tablespoons parsley, chopped
Romano cheese, grated (sheep/imported)

Place tomatoes into boiling water for 10 seconds. Peel and chop roughly (If you wish to skip this step, use a can of diced tomatoes, drained). Set tomatoes aside. Peel eggplant and then cut into 1-inch cubes. In a large skillet, heat olive oil, add garlic and onion and sauté until tender. Add eggplant, zucchini, and peppers. Fry vegetables gently (It may be necessary to add more oil). Stir in spices, salt and pepper and white wine if needed. Cover and simmer for 30 minutes. Remove lid, add tomatoes, and allow them to heat thoroughly. Sprinkle with Romano cheese and parsley.
**Serve 6 -8**

## GRILLED CHEESY ZUCCHINI

### AF (Dairy-free, Egg-free, Corn-free, Gluten-free)

3 tablespoon margarine, milk-free, corn-free
1 garlic clove, minced
6 small zucchinis, sliced
3 tablespoons parsley, chopped
½ teaspoon salt
1/8 teaspoon white pepper
6 ounces Feta cheese, crumbled (goat/imported)
1 ½ tablespoons Romano cheese, grated (sheep/imported)
3 tablespoons pimento, chopped

In large skillet, melt margarine, and sauté garlic. Add zucchini, cook until tender, and then place on greased cookie sheet. Sprinkle with parsley, salt and white pepper. Top with crumbled Feta and grated Romano cheeses. Place under broiler until lightly brown, 1 to 2 minutes. Top with pimento for color.
**Serves 6-8**

## SKILLET ZUCCHINI

### T (Testing for Dairy—Egg-free, Corn-free, Gluten-free)

4 small zucchinis
4 tablespoons margarine
1 garlic, minced
1 tablespoon paprika
¼ cup Parmesan cheese, grated
Salt and Pepper to taste

Wash and slice zucchini. Melt margarine or butter in a skillet and sauté garlic and zucchini. Cook zucchini until just tender, sprinkle with paprika and Parmesan cheese. Serve hot.
**Serves 6**

Note: To make this recipe Allergy Free simply exchange Romano cheese for the Parmesan cheese and use a margarine that is milk-free and corn-free.

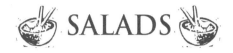

# SALADS

## TURKEY GRAPE SALAD

**(Dairy-free, Corn-free, Gluten-free)**
2 cups smoked turkey or chicken, sliced, cubed
½ teaspoon dried basil
1 cup celery, diced
1 cup red seedless grapes, sliced in half
Lettuce leaves
**Dressing:**
½ cup mayonnaise
2 tablespoons lemon juice
¼ teaspoon salt
1/8 teaspoon pepper

Mix all ingredients together and chill at least 4 hours. Serve on beds of lettuce leaves.
**Serves 4**

## ITALIAN ARTICHOKE AND TOMATO SALAD

**AF (Dairy-free, Egg-free, Corn-free, Gluten-free)**
1 fourteen ounce can artichoke hearts, chopped
1 four ounce can sliced olives
¼ cup pine nuts
2 medium tomatoes, quartered or 8 cherry tomatoes, halved
Mixed greens
¼ cup Italian dressing*
Romano cheese, grated (sheep milk)

In salad bowl, mix artichoke hearts, olives, tomatoes and pine nuts with Italian dressing. Marinate for 2 to 4 hours. Place mixture on top of mixed greens, sprinkle with Romano cheese.
**Serves 4**

## GREEK PASTA SALAD

### AF (Dairy-free, Egg-free, Corn-free, Gluten-free)

16 ounce pasta swirls, cooked and cooled
1 teaspoon Cavender's All Purpose Greek Dressing
1 cup crumbled spicy goat cheese, feta is a good choice
3 tomatoes, quartered
4 green onions, sliced
1/3 cup sun-dried tomatoes, chopped
1 seven-ounce can olives, chopped
Italian Dressing *

Cook pasta according to package instruction. Drain, cool and dry. Add a little olive oil if necessary. Mix next six ingredients into bowl with cooked pasta. Add Dressing and toss gently. Chill before serving.
**Serves 8**

## MACARONI SALAD

### T (Testing for Egg yolks—Dairy-free, Corn-free, Gluten-free)

12 ounce package rice macaroni pasta, cooked
2 tablespoon green pepper, chopped (precook in microwave for 15 seconds then cool)
1 ½ tablespoon onion, chopped (precook in microwave for 15 seconds then cool)
¾ cup celery, chopped (precook in microwave for 15 seconds then cool)
1 cup Colby goat cheddar or goat jack cheese
(found in specialty stores and some markets)
½ cup pickle relish
¾ to 1 cup Hains mayonnaise (contains egg yolk, but no egg whites).
2 tablespoons pimento, chopped
¾ teaspoon salt

Mix all ingredients together in salad bowl. Chill for about 4 hours.
**Serves 8**
> Note: Before mixing in the chopped peppers, onion, and celery cook 15 to30 seconds in microwave. Let cool. This will help the insoluble fibers of the pepper, onions, and celery to break down easier.

**SEASONED RICE SALAD**

**(Dairy-free, Corn-free, Gluten-free)**

1 to 2 cups seasoned cooked rice (see recipe below)
1 stalk celery, finely chopped
$\frac{1}{2}$ cup green pepper, finely chopped
4 green onions, finely chopped
1 four ounce jar pimento, chopped
$\frac{1}{2}$ of (14 ounce) jar of green onions
2 jars marinated artichoke hearts (reserve liquid of one jar) drained, chopped
$\frac{1}{2}$ cup mayonnaise

In a bowl, combine the rice, celery, green peppers, onions, pimento, olives, and artichokes hearts. Mix $\frac{1}{4}$ cup of liquid from artichoke heart jar with mayonnaise. Mix into salad. Chill overnight.
**Serves 8**

**Cooked Seasoned Rice:**
1 tablespoon olive oil
$\frac{1}{2}$ cup red onion, chopped
1 cup rice
2 cups chicken stock* or chicken broth
$\frac{1}{4}$ teaspoon thyme
$\frac{1}{4}$ teaspoon marjoram
$\frac{1}{4}$ teaspoon poultry seasoning

In sauce pan, heat oil. Add onions, garlic, and sauté 2 to 3 minutes. Add rice and cook one minute. Add broth and spices. Bring to broil, reduce heat. Cover with tight lid and simmer for 20 minutes. Do not check on rice until after the 20 minutes.

## ARTICHOKE HEART AND HEARTS OF PALM SALAD

### AF (Dairy-free, Egg-free, Corn-free, Gluten-free)

1 head of Boston lettuce, cleaned, broken into bite size pieces
½ head of romaine, or green lettuce (not iceberg), cleaned, broken into bite size pieces
2 seven ounce jars of marinated artichoke hearts, coarsely chopped (reserve liquid)
1 fourteen ounce can hearts of palm, sliced
2 medium tomatoes, quartered

Mix ingredients in bowl, top with Dijon Vinaigrette (recipe below). Serve on salad plates
**Serves 6**

### Dijon Vinaigrette:
1 clove garlic, minced
1/3 cup reserve liquid from marinated artichokes
1 tablespoon white wine vinegar
1 tablespoon Dijon mustard
¼ teaspoon salt
1/8 teaspoon pepper
Mix with whisk. Pour over salad.

## FETA BEET SALAD
This salad is fast, colorful and easy.

### AF (Dairy-free, Egg-free, Corn-free, Gluten-free)

1 packaged fresh beets, sliced, precooked
  (Trader Joe's and others sell them in the refrigerator section)
1 package of fresh mixed greens
1 (3.5 ounce) package feta cheese
½ cup toasted pistachio nuts, chopped

### Dressing:
¼ cup balsamic vinegar
½ cup olive oil

Mix oil and vinegar in small mixing bowl. On separate salad plates arrange mix greens. Place sliced beets on top of greens pour salad dressing over each plate of greens. Top with Feta and pistachios.
**Serves 4-6**

## GARBANZO BEAN BEET SALAD

### AF (Dairy-free, Egg-free, Corn-free, Gluten-free)

½ cup fresh beets, packaged and precooked
¼ cup green onions, sliced
½ cup celery, sliced
¼ cup sesame seed, toasted
½ cup garbanzo beans
¼ teaspoon salt
Dash pepper
Eggless mayonnaise
Mixed Greens

Mix ingredients together and chill. Serve on bed of lettuce.
**Serves 4**


## CARROT-RAISIN SALAD

### AF (Dairy-free, Egg-free, Corn-free, Gluten-free)

2 cups carrots, shredded
1 cup raisins
½ to 1 cup Eggless mayonnaise (Vegenaise)
1/3 cup honey (optional)

Mix all ingredients together and refrigerate for at least 1 hour.
**Serves 4**

## NUTTY FRUIT SALAD

### AF (Dairy-free, Egg-free, Corn-free, Gluten-free)

½ cup almonds, chopped
½ cup pitted cherries
½ cup peach, sliced in own juice or fresh
½ cup fresh or frozen cranberries, cooked
1/3 cup honey
1/3 cup Eggless mayonnaise, corn-free

In small skillet, toast almond. Set aside. Combine cherries, peaches, cranberries, and honey. Toss and chill. Serve on separate salad plates on any variety of lettuce. Top with almonds.

**Serves 4**

## AVOCADO PROVENCAL SALAD

### AF (Dairy-free, Egg-free, Corn-free, Gluten-free)

2 packages of mix greens
1 package of baby spinach
2 (14 ounce) cans of artichoke hearts
1 avocado, peeled, pitted and diced
½ cup sliced shallots
½ to 1 cup Curried Italian Dressing*
2 tablespoons parsley, chopped

Chop mixed greens and spinach into bite size pieces. Chill. Slice artichokes into 1-inch pieces. Place artichokes, olives, shallots and salad dressing into mixing bowl. Toss and chill for 2 hours before serving. Just before serving prepared avocado. Place chilled greens onto salad plates. Mix avocado with artichoke mixture and top onto greens. Sprinkle with parsley.

**Serves 6-8**

## CUCUMBER SALAD PLATTER

### AF (Dairy-free, Egg-free, Corn-free, Gluten-free)

2 large cucumbers, sliced
4 large tomatoes, sliced
1 (14 ounce) mixed olives or a mixture of olives from grocery olive bars
¼ cup peppercini rings
1 small onion, finely chopped
2 tablespoons virgin olive oil
2 tablespoon red wine vinegar
¼ teaspoon oregano
1 garlic, minced
Salt and Pepper to taste

Prepare cucumbers and tomatoes. Arrange olives and peppercinis on rimmed platter. Place chopped onion and garlic in microwave and cook for 15 seconds. Cool. Mix onions and garlic with wine vinegar, oregano, salt and pepper. Pour over vegetables, and marinate 2-3 hours before serving.

**Serves 4**

## EGGPLANT FETA SALAD

### AF (Dairy-free, Egg-free, Corn-free, Gluten-free)

1 medium eggplant
1 cup onion, chopped
4 tablespoons olive oil
2 tablespoons white wine vinegar
½ teaspoon salt
¼ teaspoon pepper
¼ cup parsley, chopped
3 medium tomatoes, sliced
1 (2.25 ounce) can olives, sliced
1 large green pepper, cut into strips
1 (3.5 ounces) Feta cheese, cubed or crumbles (sheep/imported)

Wrap whole eggplant into aluminum foil. Bake in a preheated 350 degree oven for 35 to 45 minutes. Peel off skin and cut eggplant into cubes. Microwave onion and green pepper for 15 to 30 seconds(for "IBS individuals) and cool. In a mixing bowl, combine eggplant with onion, oil, vinegar, salt and pepper. Chill for 2 hours. To serve, place on salad platter, sprinkle with parsley surround with green peppers, tomatoes, and olives. Top with Feta cheese. **Serves 8**

## SPICY SPINACH SALAD

### AF (Dairy-free, Egg-free, Corn-free, Gluten-free)

1 package baby spinach
1 package mixed greens or European greens
3 large tomatoes, cut into wedges
1 cucumber, peeled and slices
1 tablespoon capers
1 teaspoon Cavender's All Purpose Greek Seasoning
¼ cup celery, chopped
½ cup fresh wild mushroom, sliced
1 (2.25 ounce) can black olives, sliced
1 container of 3.5 ounces Feta cheese (sheep/imported)

Tear spinach and greens into bite-size pieces and arrange on a platter. Combine other ingredients, except for cheese, in a mixing bowl; then pour on top of lettuce. Crumble Feta and sprinkle on top of salad. Top with Greek Salad Dressing*.**Serves 4-6**

## ORIENTAL SPINACH-SESAME SALAD

### AF (Dairy-free, Egg-free, Corn-free, Gluten-free)

1 package of baby spinach
½ cup of sesame seeds
2 tablespoons canola oil
2 tablespoons lemon juice
2 tablespoons tamari soy sauce (organic/wheat-free)
1 teaspoon salt
¼ teaspoon hot pepper sauce
1 cup fresh mushrooms, thinly slices
1 can water chestnuts, drained and sliced

Tear spinach into bite size pieces. In medium-size saucepan, heat sesame seeds until brown. Add oil, lemon juice, tamari, salt and hot pepper sauce. Pour mixture into salad bowl. Chill for at least 1 hour. Before serving, add spinach leaves and toss well.
**Serves 4**

## PACHADI

### T (Testing for corn—Dairy-free, Egg-free, Gluten-free)

1 cup green cabbage, shredded (usually comes in 16 ounce packages)
1 cup carrots, grated
1 cup cucumber, unpeeled, sliced
2 green chili peppers, cut in slivers
½ cup shallots, chopped
1 teaspoon tamari soy sauce (organic/wheat-free)
1 cup whipped topping, dairy-free (cool whip is the best,
 second ingredient is corn syrup)
½ teaspoon paprika
1 tablespoon coriander, ground
Watercress sprigs

Combine all ingredients except watercress. Chill for 2 hours. Place mixture on top of watercress sprigs.
**Serves 4**

## PICNIC POTATO SALAD

### AF (Dairy-free, Egg-free, Corn-free, Gluten-free)

5 medium potatoes, peeled, washed and cubed
2 teaspoons salt
³⁄₄ cup celery, chopped
¹⁄₂ cup green pepper, finely chopped
¹⁄₄ cup dill pickles, chopped
2 tablespoons parsley, chopped
1 cup scallions, chopped
2 tablespoons prepared mustard
1 ¹⁄₂ cups Eggless mayonnaise (Vegenaise will work well)
Dash of paprika

Cook potatoes until tender, drain and cool for about 15 minutes. Meanwhile, pre-cook green pepper in microwave for about 15 seconds. Let cool. Mix all ingredients together in large bowl. Refrigerate for a least 2 hours before serving. Sprinkle paprika on top with sprigs of parsley.
**Serves 6**

## ROQUEFORT AND TOMATO SALAD

### AF (Dairy-free, Egg-free, Corn-free, Gluten-free)

3 medium tomatoes, cut into wedges
1 package of Mesclun lettuce mix (some stores call it the European mix)
2 tablespoons Roquefort cheese (sheep/imported)
**Dressing:**
1 tablespoons red wine vinegar
3 tablespoons olive oil
¹⁄₂ teaspoon salt
Dash of pepper

In small bowl, mix together vinegar, oil, salt and pepper. Place tomatoes in a container, pour dressing over tomatoes. Let chill 1 hour. Place tomatoes on salad plates with Mesclun, pour remaining dressing over tomatoes, and sprinkle Roquefort cheese on top.
**Serves 4**

## APPLE NUT SLAW

### AF (Dairy-free, Egg-free, Corn-free, Gluten-free)

3 cups unpeeled red apples, cored, chopped
1 cup roasted almonds, chopped
1 cup Egg-free mayonnaise
2 tablespoons lemon juice
1 tablespoon honey
1 teaspoon salt
$\frac{1}{2}$ head of butter lettuce, cleaned

In a large bowl, combine all ingredients. Chill for 1 hour before serving. Serve on beds of Butter lettuce.
**Serves 4-6**

## ZUCCHINI SALAD

### T (Testing for egg—Dairy-free, Corn-free, Gluten-free)

2 small zucchinis, sliced
2 large tomatoes, cut into wedges
$\frac{1}{4}$ head iceberg lettuce, shredded
$\frac{1}{4}$ head romaine lettuce, chopped
$\frac{1}{2}$ cup shallots, chopped
2 tablespoons parsley, chopped
1 two-ounce jar pimento, chopped
1 hard-boiled, chopped
1 garlic clove, minced
$\frac{1}{2}$ cup sesame seed oil
Salt to taste

Brush zucchini slices with oil, place them on a cookie sheet and broil until lightly brown. Dice cooked zucchini and cool. In large bowl Add zucchinis, lettuces, shallots, parsley, and pimento; toss. In separate small bowl, whisk garlic, lemon juice and sesame oil together to make dressing. When ready to serve, place on platter, garnish with chopped egg. Pour dressing over salad.
**Serves 4-6**

# DRESSINGS, GRAVIES AND SAUCES

**FRENCH DRESSING I**

**AF (Dairy-free, Egg-free, Corn-free, Gluten-free)**

1 ½ cup olive oil
½ cup tarragon vinegar
1 teaspoon salt
½ teaspoon pepper
2 teaspoons shallots, chopped
1 teaspoon paprika

Mix ingredients and refrigerate up to 2 days.
**Makes 2 cups**

**FRENCH DRESSING II**

**AF (Dairy-free, Egg-free, Corn-free, Gluten-free)**

1 cup canola or olive oil
2 tablespoons paprika
1 garlic clove, pressed
¼ cup white wine vinegar
1 teaspoon salt
2 tablespoons parsley, chopped
   dash of cayenne pepper

Combine all ingredients, mix well with a whisk, and refrigerate.
**Makes 1 ½ cups**

## GARLIC DIJON DRESSING

### AF (Dairy-free, Egg-free, Corn-free, Gluten-free)

1 large garlic clove, pressed
Squirt of Dijon mustard to taste (about ¼ teaspoon)
Pinch of dry thyme to taste
Pinch of salt and pepper to taste
3 tablespoons Almond oil
1 tablespoon canola oil
2 tablespoons white wine vinegar

Make a roux of the first four ingredients, and then add all of the oil and vinegar last. Blend well with a whisk. Refrigerate.

**Makes about ¼ cup dressing** (make this dressing in small quantities to keep the garlic flavor fresh)

## ROQUEFORT DRESSING

### AF (Dairy-free, Egg-free, Corn-free, Gluten-free)

1 cup Egg-free mayonnaise (Vegenaise is a good choice)
1/3 cup sour cream substitute (most contain soy)
¼ cup Roquefort cheese, crumbles (sheep/imported)
1 garlic clove, pressed
3 tablespoons white wine vinegar

Combine ingredients with a mixing whisk and refrigerate.
**Makes 1 ½ cups**

## DILLWEED SAUCE

### AF (Dairy-free, Egg-free, Corn-free, Gluten-free)

2 tablespoons margarine, dairy-free, corn-free
1 tablespoon chives, snipped
1 tablespoon lemon juice
1 teaspoon dill weed
½ teaspoon salt
1/8 teaspoon pepper
1 medium dill pickle, finely chopped

Melt margarine in a saucepan. Add lemon juice, salt pepper and dill weed. Mix until blended. Add chopped pickles just before serving.
**Makes ½ cup**

## EGG-FREE MAYONNAISE

### AF (Dairy-free, Egg-free, Corn-free, Gluten-free)

1 teaspoon sugar
1 teaspoon salt
¼ teaspoon paprika
1 teaspoon dry mustard
¼ cup sour cream substitute (contains soy)
1/3 cup canola oil
3 teaspoons vinegar
3 teaspoons lemon juice
2/3 cup canola oil

Mix together sugar, salt, paprika and dry mustard. Add sour cream substitute. Add 1/3 cup salad oil 1 teaspoon at a time, and beat well. In a separate bowl, mix together vinegar and lemon juice. Add this mixture alternately with the 2/3 cup of oil. Mix well after each addition. Mix both mixtures together. Cover and chill.
**Makes 1 ¼ cups**

## TARRAGON DRESSING

### AF (Dairy-free, Egg-free, Corn-free, Gluten-free)

¼ teaspoon dry tarragon
1 teaspoon salt
½ teaspoon pepper
¼ cup shallots, chopped
½ cup tarragon vinegar
1 cup olive oil
1 teaspoon Dijon-type mustard

Combine all ingredients with a whisk and refrigerate.
**Makes 1 ½ cups**

## GREEK SALAD DRESSING

### AF (Dairy-free, Egg-free, Corn-free, Gluten-free)

1 teaspoon Cavender's All Purpose Greek Seasoning
½ teaspoon oregano
½ teaspoon basil leaf, crumbled
½ teaspoon salt
¼ teaspoon pepper
2 tablespoons onion, grated
1 teaspoon Dijon-type mustard
½ cup wine vinegar
1 cup Basil-flavored olive oil (available at stores like Whole foods or Trader Joes)

Combine above ingredients with whisk and refrigerate.
**Makes 1 ½ cups**

## CURRIED ITALIAN DRESSING

**AF (Dairy-free, Egg-free, Corn-free, Gluten-free)**

1 tablespoon Italian Seasoning
4 tablespoons red wine vinegar
2 tablespoons parsley, finely chopped
1 garlic clove, pressed
½ teaspoon curry powder
2 tablespoons Dijon-type mustard
½ cup olive oil
¼ teaspoon salt
Dash of pepper

Combine above ingredients in a small bowl. Chill
**Makes ¾ cup**

## MUSHROOM SAUCE

**AF (Dairy-free, Egg-free, Corn-free, Gluten-free)**

2 tablespoons margarine, milk-free, corn-free
¾ cup of crimini mushrooms, chopped
2 tablespoon of dry or fresh shitake mushrooms
2 tablespoons white rice flour
1 tablespoon dill weed
1 teaspoon fennel seed, smashed with a mortar and pestle
2 cups chicken broth
¼ cup non-dairy creamer (or sour cream)

In a saucepan, melt margarine and sauté mushrooms until tender (Note: with dry mushrooms they must be soaked in **HOT** water for 20 minutes first). Stir in rice flour, and then slowly add chicken broth. Add dill weed and fennel seed. Cover and simmer for 20 minutes or until thickened. Remove from heat and add creamer. Non-dairy sour cream can be used instead of creamer. It usually contains soy.
**Makes 2 ¼ cups**

## CILANTRO DRESSING

### AF (Dairy-free, Egg-free, Corn-free, Gluten-free)

$1/2$ cup mayonnaise substitute (I used Vegenaise)
3 green onions sliced
$1/2$ cup to 1 cup cilantro, washed, stems removed

In small food processor, chop cilantro and green onions. Add mayonnaise substitute. Mix until smooth.
**Makes $1/2$ cup**

## CHIPOTLE DRESSING

### AF (Dairy-free, Egg-free, Corn-free, Gluten-free)

$1/2$ cup mayonnaise substitute
1 teaspoon chipotle chili in adobo sauce (remove seeds to decrease heat, using vinyl gloves)
2 teaspoons adobo sauce

In small food processor, chop chilies and sauce. Add mayonnaise substitute. Mix until smooth.
**Makes $1/2$ cups**

176

## ASIAN CRANBERRY SAUCE
Fresh cranberries are difficult to find in the summer. Rehydrating dried cranberries works well.

**AF (Dairy-free, Egg –free, Corn-free, Gluten-free)**

1 2/3 cup or 6 ounce package of dried cranberries, sweetened
2 cups water
1 tablespoon Hoisin Sauce
2 tablespoons orange juice
1 teaspoon Chinese 5 spices

Place cranberries in saucepan with water. Heat pan until boiling, reduce heat and simmer for 5 minutes. Remove pan from heat and allow cranberries and liquid to cool. Drain cranberries through a sieve. Reserve cranberry water and set aside. In food processor or blender, place drained cranberries, Hoisin Sauce, Chinese 5 spices, orange juice and 1/8 to ¼ cup of reserved boiled liquid. Pulse until mixture is desired texture.
**Makes 1 ¼ cups sauce.**

## SPICY TOMATO KETCHUP

**AF (Dairy-free, Corn-free, Egg-free, Gluten-free)**

2/3 cup tomato sauce
3 tablespoons tomato paste
1 teaspoon apple cider vinegar
1 to 2 tablespoons sugar
½ teaspoon onion salt
Dash to 1/8 teaspoon cinnamon
Dash cayenne pepper

Mix ingredients together in bowl. Chill.
**Makes 1 cup**

**SPICY BARBECUE SAUSE**

**AF (Dairy-free, Egg-free, Corn-free, Gluten-free)**

½ cup Spicy Tomato Ketchup
1 tablespoon molasses
2 tablespoons brown sugar
3 teaspoons Worcestershire sauce
½ teaspoon Smoked Hickory Seasoning
½ teaspoon garlic powder
1/8 teaspoon cayenne pepper

Mix ingredients together in mixing bowl. Refrigerate until use.
**Makes ¾ cup**


**BOUQUET GARNI**

Tie up in cheesecloth:
6 sprigs parsley
6 basil leaves
3 garlic cloves, unpeeled, slightly crushed
1 large bay leaf
7 peppercorns


**PREPARED MISO SAUCE**

**AF (Dairy-free, Egg-free, Corn-free, Gluten-free)**

1 cup water
4 ounces rice miso
1 tablespoon soy sauce (organic/wheat-free)

In saucepan, over low heat, add water to miso and tamari. Stir until you have a smooth sauce. Do not overheat. Refrigerate.
**Makes 1 ¼ cups**

## HEADACHE-FREE SEASONED SALT

### AF (Dairy-free, Egg-free, Corn-free, Gluten-free)

4 teaspoons Italian seasoning
2 teaspoons turmeric
4 teaspoons garlic salt (be careful to read label)
4 teaspoons onion salt
2 teaspoons paprika
2 teaspoons potato starch

Mix seasonings. Store mixture in a sealed container.

## BEEF GRAVY

### AF (Dairy-free, Egg-free, Corn-free, Gluten-free)

$\frac{1}{2}$ cube margarine, milk-free, corn-free
1/3 cup carrots, chopped
$\frac{1}{2}$ cup onion, chopped
1 celery rib, chopped
2 tablespoon white rice flour
2 tablespoon cooked beef, finely chopped (optional)
1 cup chicken broth
3 cups beef broth
1 bay leaf
$\frac{1}{2}$ teaspoon thyme
Salt and Pepper to taste

Melt margarine in large saucepan. Add carrots, onions, and celery; sauté till tender. Add rice flour and mix with vegetables. Slowly add chicken broth to saucepan so not to avoid any lumps. Add beef broth, chopped beef, thyme, bay leaf, salt and pepper. Bring mixture to boil, reduce heat and simmer covered for 20 minutes. Strain gravy through sieve into another saucepan, removing bay leaf, and vegetable mixture. (At this point, gravy can be refrigerated and stored up to a week.) Return gravy to heat. Add 1 tablespoon arrowroot dissolved in $\frac{1}{4}$ cup water to gravy to thicken. Heat gravy for 5 to 10 minutes.
**Makes approximately 3 $\frac{1}{2}$ cups**

## TURKEY /CHICKEN GRAVY

This is great gravy for Thanksgiving. You may want to double the recipe.

**AF (Dairy-free, Egg-free, Corn-free, Gluten-free)**

1/3 cup carrots, chopped
$\frac{1}{2}$ cup onions, chopped
1 celery rib
$\frac{1}{2}$ cube margarine, milk-free, corn-free
2 tablespoons white rice flour
1 cup beef broth
3 cups chicken broth
  drippings from turkey or chicken (maybe added at any time)
1 bay leaf
$\frac{1}{2}$ teaspoon thyme
$\frac{1}{4}$ teaspoon sage
$\frac{1}{4}$ teaspoon poultry seasoning
  salt and pepper to taste

Melt margarine in large saucepan. Add carrots, onions, and celery; sauté until tender. Add rice flour and mix with vegetables. Slowly add beef broth to avoid any lumps. Add chicken broth, drippings (if available), bay leaf, spice, salt and pepper. Heat to boiling, reduce heat and simmer for 20 minutes. Remove pan from heat and pour gravy through a strainer into another saucepan. This will remove the vegetables and bay leaf. (At this point the gravy may be stored and refrigerated up to a week.) Return gravy to heat. Add 1 tablespoon arrowroot mixed with $\frac{1}{4}$ cup water to gravy to thicken. Heat 5 to 10 minutes more.
**Makes approximately 3 $\frac{1}{2}$ cup gravy**

# CAKES, PIES & DESSERTS

## APPLE CAKE

### Test for Eggs (Dairy-free, Corn-free Gluten-free)

1 cup rice flour
½ cup almond flour*
1 tablespoon tapioca flour
1 teaspoon baking powder
1 teaspoon baking soda
½ teaspoon salt
2 eggs, lightly beaten
1 ¼ cup sugar
½ cup vegetable oil (canola)
¼ cup orange juice
1 teaspoon vanilla extract
3 apples (Granny Smith, Fuji, Graven Stein)
1 ½ teaspoon lemon juice
1 teaspoon ground cinnamon
Powdered sugar

Preheat oven to 350 degrees. Pam a baking pan measuring 7 by 11. Sift all dry ingredients and set aside. In separate bowl, beat eggs with 1 cup sugar, add oil, orange juice and vanilla extract. Mix well. Stir egg mixture into dry ingredients until it forms a batter; do not over-mix. Set aside while preparing apples.

Core, but do not peel apples, slice thinly and toss with lemon juice, remaining sugar and cinnamon. Spoon half of the batter into the pan, layer with ½ of the apples. Spoon remaining batter on top ( but do not scrape the bowl). Make another layer of remaining apples and then scrape the bowl and dot the batter on top of the apples.

Place in oven and bake for about 45 minutes. The cake is done when a skewer is poked into it and comes out clean. Allow the cake to sit in pan. Apple juices will soak into the cake to form a moist cake. Dust with powdered sugar. A dollop of cool whip may be added but this contains corn syrup.

## CARROT CAKE

Since this cake does not rise too much, I elected to cut it in half and frost in between layers.

### (Diary-free, Corn-free, Gluten-free)

2/3 cup white rice flour
½ cup brown rice flour
1/3 cup sorghum flour     } or 1 3/4 cup of Terry's Flour Blend
2 tablespoons potato starch
2 tablespoons tapioca flour
1 teaspoon xanthan gum
1 ½ teaspoon baking powder
1 teaspoon baking soda
½ teaspoon salt
1 teaspoon cinnamon                 ½ cup canola oil
1 1/8 to 1 ¼ cup carrots, grated    2 eggs, beaten
½ cup raisins                       ¾ cup pineapple juice
1 cup sugar                         1 teaspoon vanilla

In a very large mixing bowl, mix first 5 ingredients together. Remove ¼ cup of mixed flours and put aside. Mix in xanthan gun and baking powder, soda, salt and cinnamon. In separate small bowl, mix eggs, oil, and vanilla. Add to dry mixture. Add pineapple juice. Using electric mixer, mix well (Gluten-free flours need to be mixed with a beater). Slowly add sugar. If mixture seems too thin at this point, add the extra flour. Otherwise finish by adding the rest of the ingredients, folding in raisins and carrots. Pour mixture into greased 9 by 13 baking dish. Bake at 350 degrees for 35 to 40 minutes. If cake starts to look a little too brown toward the end of the cooking time, cover with aluminum foil. Allow to cool. Cut cake in half. Top bottom layer with Cream Cheese frosting*(to follow). Place next layer on top and frost top layer. Allow to chill in refrigerator for at least 4 hours before serving.
**Serves 8-12**

### Cream Cheese Frosting

5 ounces imitation plain cream cheese, softened (contains soy)
1 cube margarine, melted, milk-free, corn-free
1 teaspoon vanilla
2 ½ cups powdered sugar

In mixing bowl, beat margarine, vanilla, and imitation cream cheese together. Slowly add powdered sugar. Mix until smooth.

## SOURCREAM GINGERBREAD

While this recipe may say it is testing for Dairy, many individuals that all allergic are not bothered by cooked or baked Dairy products. So this may not be a telling test.

**T (Testing for Dairy—Egg-free\*\*, Corn-free, Gluten-free)**

2/3 cup white rice flour
½ cup brown rice flour
1/3 cup sorghum flour          **} or 1 3/4 cup of Terry's Flour Blend**
2 tablespoons potato starch
2 tablespoons tapioca flour
1 teaspoon xanthan gum
1 ½ teaspoon baking soda
1 teaspoon cinnamon
½ teaspoon ginger
½ teaspoon cloves (optional)
¼ teaspoon salt
2/3 cup sugar
1 cube butter or margarine
2 egg whites, beaten
¾ cup blackstrap molasses
¾ cup sour cream
2/3 cup very hot water

In small bowl, mix first 5 flours together. Remove ¼ cup and set aside. Add to flour mixture the xanthan gum, baking soda, spices and salt. Meanwhile, soften butter in large bowl, cream sugar and butter together. Add molasses and egg whites to sugar mixture. Alternately add flours mixture and hot water to sugar mixture 1/3 at a time until batter is smooth. If too thin add extra ¼ cup flour that is set aside. Fold in sour cream into batter. Pour batter into greased 9 by 9 by 2 inch baking pan. Bake gingerbread at 350 degrees for 35 to 40 minutes, or until gingerbread is firm and springy to touch.
**Serves 6-8**

## CHOCOLATE WHISKEY CAKE

This cake is corn and wheat free- sort of. Whiskey contains wheat and bourbon contains corn. I am going on the theory that the alcohol will be cooked off and the protein then rendered harmless.

### (Corn-free, Gluten-free)

¼ cup scotch whiskey, or bourbon
¼ teaspoon alcohol-free almond extract
¼ cup raisins
7 ounce semi-sweet or bittersweet chocolate (about 60-70 percent pure chocolate)
½ cup unsalted butter or margarine (at room temperature and cut into pieces)
3 large eggs
½ cup sugar
4 tablespoons Terry's flour blend
2/3 cup almond flour (or ground, blanched almonds)
Pinch of salt
¼ teaspoon cream of tartar
2 tablespoons sugar

Cut up chocolate and allow to melt very slowly with butter (or margarine) and 3 tablespoons water in a small bowl placed in a pan of not quite simmering water. Sir form time to time until melted and smooth. Set aside.

Put raisins to steep in whiskey with almond extract and set aside. Separate eggs; place whites in a bowl of electric mixer and set aside; place yolks in a separate bowl with ½ cup sugar.

Whisk yolks and sugar together until creamy and pale yellow. Whisk in chocolate mixture, then flour mixture and almond flour (or ground almonds), and finally raisins, whiskey and almond extract. Set aside.

Beat egg whites with salt until foamy, then add cream of tartar and beat until soft peaks are formed, sprinkle in the 2 tablespoons sugar and continue to beat until peaks are firm and glossy.

Fold about 1/3 of the beaten whites in to the chocolate batter to lighten it. Then fold in the remaining whites quickly and gently using a cutting motion with a rubber spatula. Turn batter into pan (which has been buttered, and lined with a circle of buttered waxed or parchment paper), distribute batter evenly and bake 30-40 minutes (in a preheat oven of 375 degrees) or until cake is done around the edges (but it will remain quite moist and seemingly underdone in the center). Allow cake to cool in pan.

Turn cake out onto serving platter and continue with following options:
1. Sprinkle with powdered sugar
2. Serve with whipped topping
3. Glaze with 6 ounce semi-sweet baking chocolate melted with
   2 tablespoons butter or margarine.

## HEAVENLY CHOCOLATE MOUSSE

### (Dairy-free, Gluten-free)

¾ cup semisweet chocolate chips (60% is best)
1 (12.3 oz) package of extra-firm tofu
¼ teaspoon salt
3 large eggs whites
½ cup sugar
¼ cup water
Cool Whip (optional) contains corn syrup
Grated chocolate (optional)

Melt chocolate chips in microwave. Place melted chocolate chips and tofu in food processor. Process 2 minutes or until smooth. Place salt and egg whites in a cold medium bowl, beat with mixer at high speed until stiff peaks form. (The best bowl for beating egg whites is a copper bowl. Refrigerate the bowl)

Combine sugar and water in small saucepan, bring to a boil. Cook, without stirring, until candy thermometer registers 238. Pour the hot sugar syrup in a thin stream over the egg whites beating at high speed (this is an Italian meringue). Gently stir one-fourth of the meringue into the tofu mixture, gently fold in remaining meringue. Spoon ½ cupfuls mousse into dessert bowls. Cover and chill for at least 4 hours before serving. If desired, garnish with Cool Whip and grated chocolate.
**Serves 8**
**Variations:** Add 1 tablespoon of grand Marnier, or rum liquor to processed tofu and chocolate chips.

185

## JOANNE'S PEARS IN RED WINE

My friend Joanne delights company every time she brings this dessert.

### AF (Dairy-free, Egg-free, Corn-free, Gluten-free)

1 ¾ cups dry red wine
1 cup sugar
¼ teaspoon anise seeds

6 firm-ripe medium Bosc pears
2 to 3 thin lemons slices
2 whole cinnamon sticks

In a large Dutch oven, combine wine, sugar, anise, cinnamon sticks, and lemon slices. Bring mixture to a boil. Peel pears. Set pears into boiling mixture (make sure the pears are in one layer), and reduce heat to medium. Cover and simmer pears until pears can be pierced easily with a fork (about 15 minutes). Turn fruit occasionally so all sides of the pears are in syrup. With a slotted spoon, lift pears form syrup and transfer to a serving dish. With remaining syrup bring to boil until the liquid is reduced to ¾ to 1 cup of liquid. Pour hot syrup over and around pears. Serve warm or at room temperature.

**Serves 6**

## NEL'S SWEDISH SPONGE CAKE

### (Dairy-free, Gluten-free)

4 eggs, separated (room temperature)
1 cup sugar
½ cup potato starch
1 teaspoon baking powder (featherweight is gluten-free)
1 cup non-dairy whipped topping
½ cup chocolate shavings (semi-sweet only)
¼ cup roasted almonds, chopped

Beat eggs in cold copper bowl until stiff but not dry, then fold in ½ cup of the sugar. In separate bowl beat egg yolks and remaining sugar together. Mix yolk mixture and beaten egg whites together gently. Add potato starch and baking powder. Pour into 2 greased and floured (using sorghum flour) 8 inch pans. Bake in pre-heated oven at 350 degrees for 20 minutes. Let cool and remove from pans. Fill and top with non-dairy topping. Sprinkle with chocolate shavings and nuts. This is a delicious heirloom recipe.

**Serves 8**

**Variation:** Top non-dairy topping with 1 cup of sliced strawberries instead of chocolate and nuts.

## APPLE CRISP

### AF (Dairy-free, Egg-free, Corn-free, Gluten-free)

4 apples, cored, peeled, and sliced
2 tablespoons margarine, milk-free, corn-free
1 teaspoon cinnamon
½ cup brown sugar

1 teaspoon lemon juice
1 tablespoon sorghum flour
1 cup rolled oats, uncooked

Place sliced apples in a greased 8 by 8 inch baking dish. Sprinkle with lemon juice. Mix rest of the ingredients in a small mixing bowl and sprinkle over the apples. Bake in a pre-heated oven at 350 degrees for 20 minutes or until just golden brown. Serve warm.

**Variations:** If using fresh peach or cherries increase brown sugar to ¾ cup.

**Serves 6**

## BROWN BETTY

This is another apple crisp but using bread crumbs instead of oats.

### AF (Dairy-free, Egg-free**, Corn-free, Gluten-free)

2 cups rice bread crumbs
2 tablespoons lemon juice
½ teaspoon cinnamon
4 cups apples, cored, peeled, and chopped
2 tablespoons margarine, milk-free, corn-free
2 tablespoon margarine, cut into small squares (for topping)

1/8 teaspoon salt
¼ teaspoon nutmeg
2 tablespoons water
¾ cup sugar

Melt margarine in microwave. In small bowl, mix bread crumbs with melted margarine. Mix sugar and spices in separate bowl. Grease 9 by 13 baking dish. Place ¼ of bread crumb mixture in the baking dish. Top with ½ of the chopped apples followed by sprinkling ¼ of sugar mixture. Add another ¼ of crumb mixture top with rest of the apples and rest of the sugar mixture. Mix water and lemon juice together pour over layered apples. Place rest of crumbs on top. Dot the remaining margarine on top of the crumbs. Cover with foil and bake in pre-heat oven at 375 degrees for 45 minutes. Uncover and allow to brown, approximately 5 minutes. Serve with non-dairy topping.

**Serves 8**

## PUMPKIN CHIFFON PIE

### T (Testing for eggs—Dairy-free, Corn-free, Gluten-free)

3 eggs, separated
3/4 cup brown sugar
1 1/2 cup canned pumpkin
1/2 teaspoon salt
1 teaspoon cinnamon
1 envelope unflavored gelatin

6 tablespoons sugar
1/2 cup cold water
1/2 cup rice milk
1/2 teaspoon ground ginger
1/2 teaspoon nutmeg

Baked 8 inch pie shell
Whipped topping (optional) can contain corn or soy
Beat egg yolks and brown sugar until thick; add pumpkin, milk, salt and spices. Cook mixture in double boiler until thick. Meanwhile, let gelatin stand 5 minutes in cold water, then stir into hot mixture. When dissolved, cool mixture until it begins to set. Beat egg whites until fluffy and gradually add the 6 tablespoons sugar, beating until quite stiff. Fold egg white mixture into pumpkin mixture. Pour into baked pie crust and chill. Serve with whipped topping.

### Pie Crust:
3/4 cup rice flour
1 tablespoon potato starch
1/2 teaspoon baking powder
1 1/2 tablespoon sugar
1/4 teaspoon salt
1/2 teaspoon xanthan gum
1 egg beaten
4 tablespoons margarine, milk-free, corn-free

Preheat oven to 425 degrees. Place aside a 8 inch pie pan. In medium bowl, beat egg and margarine. In another bowl, mix rice flour, potato starch, baking powder, sugar and salt. Add to egg mixture. Gently stir until blended. Place on rice floured parchment paper. Sprinkle rice flour over mixture and cover with another piece of parchment paper. Will rolling pin roll out dough larger than the pie pan. Fold the dough over on the parchment paper. Place on one half of the pie pan. Now unroll the other piece. Seal edges with finger tips. Bake at 20 minutes on lowest rack in oven.

## OLD FASHION APPLE PIE

As far as I am concerned, apple pies are labor intensive. But the results are worth it.

### AF (Dairy-free, Egg-free**, Corn-free, Gluten-free)

**Pie Filling:**
3 Granny apples, peeled and cored
3 Golden Delicious, peeled and cored
1 cup sugar
2 tablespoons sweet rice flour
½ teaspoon cinnamon
¼ teaspoon nutmeg
¼ teaspoon allspice
¼ teaspoon salt
2 teaspoons lemon juice

### 2 pie crust:
½ cup sorghum flour
½ cup potato starch
1 cup tapioca flour
¼ cup brown rice flour
½ cup white rice flour
3 tablespoons sugar
2/3 cup shortening, use smart balance or spectrum
2 tablespoons margarine, milk-free, corn-free
1/3 cup milk substitute
¼ cup ice cold water

In food processor with plastic blade, place crust ingredients, except for ice water. When placing shortening and margarine, make sure these are in small pieces. Process the ingredients until crumbly. Remove from food processor and place mixture into medium stainless steel bowl. Add ice water a little at a time. Press the dough against the bowl with spatula or wooden spoon to work the water into the dough. Remove dough when it is wet to touch and slides down the side of the bowl. Divide dough in half. Form dough into balls and flatten. Wrap in plastic wrap, and refrigerate for 1 hour or more.

As I stated before, making pies are labor intensive. This is a good place to stop and finish pie the next day.

While dough is in the refrigerator start to prepare the filling. Peel and core the apples. Cut apples into ¼ inch thick slices. Mix flour, sugar, spices, salt and lemon together with apples. Set aside.

After the hour or more, remove dough from refrigerator. Preheat oven to 425 degrees. Have pie pan ready for pie. Place dough on parchment paper with rice flour on it. Place more rice flour on top of dough. Top with another piece of parchment paper. With a rolling pin, roll the bottom dough larger than the pan. Place into pan by folding dough with the parchment paper against itself. Place ½ of the rolled dough into the pie pan. Unfold the opposite side and place in pan. Place apple filling into the pie pan. Height of apples slices should be no more than 2 inches. Do not add any liquid that may have formed. Top with 2nd pie crust using same method. Create a fluted edge to seal both top and bottom dough. Cut vents in top of top pie crust. Brush egg whites on dough. Bake at 425 on lowest oven rack for 15 minutes. Reduce heat to 375 and move pie to middle rack in oven. Cook for another 25-30 minutes. Allow to cool before serving.

**Serves 8**

# COOKIES, TREATS, AND CANDIES

## VERY CHOCOLATE FUDGY BROWNIES

### (Diary-free, Corn-free, Gluten-free)

1 cup sugar
2 large eggs
1 tablespoon hot water
2 teaspoon instant coffee granules (use decaffeinated or espresso for less caffeine)
½ cup margarine, melted (corn-free)
1 teaspoon vanilla extract
1/3 cup almond flour*
½ cup rice flour
2 tablespoons tapioca flour
2/3 cup unsweetened cocoa
¼ teaspoon salt
   powdered sugar (optional)

Preheat oven to 325 degrees. Place sugar and eggs in large bowl, beat with a mixer at high speed until thick and pale (3- 5 minutes). Combine hot water and coffee granules, stirring until coffee granules dissolve. Add coffee mixture, margarine, and vanilla extract to sugar mixture, beat at low speed until combined. Add dry ingredients and fold gradually into sugar mixture, stirring until just moist. Spread batter into 8 inch square pan sprayed with pam. Bake at 325 for 25 minutes or until the brownies spring back when touched lightly in the center. Cool in pan on a rack. Garnish with powdered sugar.

Almond flour* if almond flour is unavailable, one can use almond meal and put it into a food processor to make the flour constantancy.

## BANANA-NUT OATMEAL COOKIES

### AF (Dairy-free, Egg-free**, Corn-free, Gluten-free)

2 ripe bananas, mashed
½ cup (1 stick) margarine, melted, milk-free, corn-free
2 ½ cups rolled oats
3 tablespoons Terry's flour blend
1 teaspoon xanthan gum
½ teaspoon salt
½ teaspoon cinnamon
¼ cup almonds, chopped
¾ cup brown sugar
2 teaspoons baking powder, gluten-free
2 egg whites beaten

Mash bananas in separate bowl. Melt margarine add egg whites and mix. Add brown sugar, xanthan gum, salt, and cinnamon. Blend in oats and almonds. Drop by rounded tablespoons on an ungreased cookie sheet. Bake at 350 degrees for 15 to 20 minutes.
**Makes 3 ½ dozen**


## LACE COOKIES

### T (Testing for gluten—Dairy-free, Egg-free**, Corn-free)

2 tablespoons margarine
½ cup flour
1 ½ cups brown sugar
½ cup sugar
1 teaspoon vanilla
1 teaspoon baking powder

½ cup almonds, roasted, chopped
2 egg whites, beaten

Soften margarine in microwave. Cream margarine with vanilla and sugars; add eggs and mix together well. Add baking powder to flour. Add to sugar mixture. Fold in chopped almonds. Chill 30 minutes. Drop with teaspoon on greased cookie sheet. Bake at 400 degrees for 8 minutes.
**Makes 2 dozen cookies**

## PISTACHIO BROWN SUGAR COOKIES

### AF (Dairy-free, Egg-free**, Corn-free, Gluten-free)

3 tablespoons margarine
2/3 cup brown sugar
1 ¾ cup gluten-free baking mix (either mine or commercial brand)
1 ½ teaspoons baking powder, gluten-free
1 teaspoon xanthan gum
2 egg whites (to be used separately)
½ cup pistachio nuts

In separate bowl, cream sugar and margarine. Add 1 of the egg whites. Mix in baking mix, xanthan gum, and baking powder. Mix well. Roll into small balls. Place on a greased cookie sheet about 1 inch apart. Flatten dough with fork. Brush with egg white and top with nuts. Bake in 400 degree oven for 10 minutes.
**Makes 1 ½ dozen**


## MERINGUE COOKIES

### AF (Dairy-free, Egg-free**, Corn-free, Gluten-free)

2 egg whites (room temperature)
½ teaspoon cream of tartar
¾ cup sugar
½ cup almonds, chopped

Beat egg whites until stiff but not dry. Add cream of tartar. Slowly beat in sugar, add almonds. Drop mixture onto a cookie sheet lined with wax paper. Bake in preheated oven at 275 degrees. Put cookies into oven, and turn off heat. Do not open oven or remove cookies until the next morning.
**Makes 1 ½ dozen**

## CHOCOLATE MERINGUE COOKIES

### AF (Dairy-free, Egg-free**, Corn-free, Gluten-free)

3 egg whites
½ cup sugar
1/3 cup unsweetened chocolate, grated
1 teaspoon vanilla

Beat egg whites until stiff but not dry. Add vanilla. Slowly beat in sugar. Fold in grated chocolate. Drop mixture onto greased cookie sheet. Bake in a very slow oven, about 250 to 275 degrees for 45 minutes.
**Makes 1 ½ dozen**

## SOFT MOLASSES COOKIES

### T (Testing for gluten—Dairy-free, Egg-free, Corn-free)

1 cup blackstrap molasses
1 teaspoon cream of tartar
1 cup sugar
1 ½ cups margarine, milk-free, corn-free
3 tablespoon water
2 teaspoons baking powder
3 tablespoons canola oil
2 teaspoons baking soda
4 cups flour
1 cup water
1 teaspoon ginger
1 teaspoon salt

Mix together molasses and margarine, add cream of tartar and sugar. In separate bowl, beat together oil, water and baking powder. Add this mixture to molasses mixture. Sir in baking soda, flour, water, ginger, and salt. Chill mixture for 2 hours. Drop on a cookie sheet with a spoon and bake at 375 degrees for 8 to 12 minutes.
**Makes 5 dozen**

## CHERRY PISTACHIO OATMEAL COOKIES

**AF (Dairy-free, Egg-free\*\*, Corn-free, Gluten-free)**

2/3 cup white rice flour
½ cup brown rice flour
1/3 cup sorghum flour     } **or 1 3/4 cup of Terry's Flour Blend**
2 tablespoons Potato starch
2 tablespoons Tapioca flour
1 teaspoon xanthan gum
1 teaspoon baking powder
1 teaspoon baking soda
1 teaspoon cinnamon
½ teaspoon nutmeg
¼ teaspoon salt
½ cup sugar
½ cup brown sugar
1 ½ cubes margarine, milk-free, corn-free
3 cups quick cooking rolled oats
½ cup salted pistachio nuts, shelled, skin removed and chopped\*
1 cup dried cherries
2 egg whites, beaten
6-8 ounces pineapple juice

In separate small bowl, place cherries. Pour approximately 1 cup boiling water over cherries and allow them to plump up. Drain cherries through sieve and set aside. Mix first 5 flours together in small bowl. Remove ¼ cup of combination and set aside. Add baking powder, baking soda, xanthan gum, spices and salt. In large bowl, soften margarine; add both sugars and beat with mixer until creamy. Mix egg whites into sugar mixture. Alternately add flour mixture and pineapple juice until smooth batter. If batter looks to thin, add the ¼ cup of flour sitting aside. Add cherries and pistachio nuts. Fold in oats. Drop cookies on ungreased cookie sheet. Cook at 400 degrees for 12-15 minutes.

**Makes 5 dozen cookies**
\*Note: If pistachio nuts are unsalted then add ¼ teaspoon more salt.

## ORANGE CORNMEAL COOKIES

These cookies have an interesting texture to them.

### T (Testing for citrus—Dairy-free, Gluten-free)

¾ cup brown sugar
1/3 cup honey
1 egg, beaten
½ cup almond meal
2 tablespoon potato starch
1/3 cup margarine, milk-free,
   corn-free, melted
   confectioners' Sugar

¼ cup soy flour
1 cup cornmeal
1 teaspoon vanilla
2 tablespoon orange juice
2 tablespoons grated orange rind

In small bowl, mix almond meal, cornmeal and soy flour together. In a separate bowl, blend together brown sugar, honey, vanilla and melted margarine. Add egg beat well. Mix in orange juice and orange rind. Slowly add flour mixture. If batter is too thick add more orange juice. Drop cookies on a greased cookie sheet. Bake at 375 degrees for 12-15 minutes. Sprinkle Confectioners' sugar over each cookie when cooled.

**Serves 8**

## ALMOND TOFFEE

### AF (Dairy-free, Egg-free, Corn-free, Gluten-free)

1 cup almonds, roasted and chopped
1 cup brown sugar
1 cube plus 2 tablespoons margarine, milk-free, corn free
5 ounces 60% chocolate, organic, semi-sweet

Grease with margarine, small jelly roll pan. Spread chopped almonds on bottom of pan. Dissolve sugar into butter. Bring mixture to boil, reduce to simmer for 5 to 6 minutes or until candy thermometer registers 127 degrees C. The mixture needs to be stirred the entire time. Meanwhile, melt chocolate in microwave. Pour sugar mixture into pan. Spread melted chocolate over mixture. Chill and cut into squares.

**Makes 2 ½ dozen candies**

# BEVERAGES

## APPLE-BANANA DRINK

### AF (Dairy-free, Egg-free, Corn-free, Gluten-free)

2 bananas, mashed
1 apple, cored, peeled, chopped
2 cup apple juice, pure
¼ cup honey

Place all ingredients in a blender or food processor and blend until smooth. Chill and serve.
**Makes 2 ¼ cups**


## COOL BANANA PICKUP

### AF (Dairy-free, Egg-free, Corn-free, Gluten-free)

2 medium bananas, mashed
2 cups milk substitute, soy milk is best
1/3 cup honey

Mix together in a blender or food processor. Chill
**Makes 2 cups**


## TOFU COCONUT MILK

### AF (Dairy-free, Egg-free, Corn-free, Gluten-free)

2 cups silken tofu, mashed
2 cups grated unsweetened coconut
½ cup honey
2 teaspoons vanilla

Put all ingredients in a blender or food processor and blend until smooth. Pour through a sieve lined with cheesecloth. Chill 3 hours.
**Makes 2 cups**

## VEGETABLE COCKTAIL

### AF (Dairy-free, Egg-free, Corn-free, Gluten-free)

1 medium cucumber, peeled, grated
½ cup carrots, grated
2 cups tomato juice
2 tablespoons scallions, chopped
1 teaspoon miso
1 teaspoon salt
2 drops hot pepper sauce
Dash cayenne pepper
Garnish parsley

Into blender or food processor, place all ingredients, except parsley. (Note: if you do not want to grate carrots and cucumber place in food processor first for 2 pulses, then add rest of ingredients). Run blender on puree or pulse processor for at least 6 pulses. Strain through a sieve lined with cheesecloth. Chill. Serve with sprinkles of parsley.
**Makes 2 ¼ cups**

## STRAWBERRY RASPBERRY SMOOTHIE

### AF (Dairy-free, Egg-free, Corn-free, Gluten-free)

2 cups frozen strawberries in sugar syrup, thawed
1 cup frozen raspberries, thawed
1 tablespoon honey
1 container silken tofu

Combine all ingredients in blender or food processor. Puree until smooth. Serve Chilled.

## GINGER BANANA PAPAYA SMOOTHIE

### AF (Dairy-free, Egg-free, Corn-free, Gluten-free)

1 cup papaya, peeled, seeded and chopped
1 banana, smashed
1 container silken tofu
$\frac{1}{2}$ cup orange juice
$\frac{1}{2}$ cup soy milk, vanilla
$\frac{1}{4}$ cup brown sugar
1 tablespoon fresh ginger, grated
1 tablespoon honey

In a food processor, puree papaya and banana together. Add silken tofu, orange juice, soy milk, brown sugar, ginger, and honey. Whip until smooth. Serve chilled

## MANGO PAPAYA SMOOTHIE

### AF (Dairy-free, Egg-free, Corn-free, Gluten-free)

8 ounces pure mango fruit juice
$\frac{1}{2}$ papaya, peeled, sliced, and seeded
$\frac{1}{4}$ cup soy milk, vanilla
$\frac{1}{2}$ teaspoon honey
3 -4 ice cubes, crushed
Place all ingredients into blender or food processor. Whip until smooth.
**Makes 1 $\frac{1}{4}$ cups**

## GINGER CARROT DRINK
This drink is refreshing without being too sweet.

### AF (Dairy-free, Egg-free, Corn-free, Gluten-free)

9 ounces pure carrot juice
$\frac{1}{4}$ cup pineapple juice
$\frac{1}{2}$ teaspoon finely grated fresh ginger
3 – 4 crushed ice cubes
Place in blender. Whip until smooth.
**Makes 1 $\frac{1}{4}$ cups**

# ✳APPENDIX A✳

**SUBSTITUTES**

The following list is just some of the substitutes available. Others not on this list may be available in your area. Read the label to make sure that other off limit foods are not in the substitutes.

**EGGS**

Ener-g Egg Substitute

Gold Harvest Egg Replacer

1 teaspoon unflavored gelatin + 3 tablespoons cold water + 2 tablespoons and 1 teaspoon boiling water

1.5 tablespoons oil + 1.5 tablespoons water + 1 teaspoon baking powder (gluten-free / egg free)

Watch out for the ingredients: albumin, ovalbumin, egg, egg products.

Egg whites (this book is looking more for egg yolk problems than problems relating to egg whites)

**CORN**

Using the same substitutes for wheat will work for corn. Watch out for ingredients: corn zein, maize and corn syrup and corn starch. Unfortunately corn starch is in EVERYTHING!

**MILK (DAIRY PRODUCTS)**

Soy milk- various brands (some may contain corn syrup)

Rice milk

Almond Milk

Goat, Ewe's, Buffalo milk cheeses

Tofu-sour creams, silken, cream cheese substitutes (cooking with tofu produces good results)

Watch out for the ingredients: whey,

**WHEAT (GLUTEN)**

I found no less than 250 wheat-free items; this is just a partial list:

| | | |
|---|---|---|
| Rice chips | Almond nut thins | Wheat-free pretzels |
| Corn tortillas | WF cereals | Fig Newman's WF (contains barley) |

| | | |
|---|---|---|
| Basmati Rice | Rice Pasta | Chunky Chocolate cookies WF |
| Sushi Rice | Rice Crisps | Buckwheat berry waffles |
| Ginger cookies | Almond Balls | Rice Thins |
| Crackers WF | Corn Pizza | Sesame and Blueberry bars |
| Lasagna pasta | Quinoa flakes | Chicken Nuggets WF (frozen) |
| Soy pudding | Rice Bread | Frozen cookie mix WF |
| Pizza mix | Frozen taquitos | Pancake/ Waffle mix |
| Amy's soups | Amy's frozen entrees | |

Note: The rice pasta deserves a special note. De Boles, Tiinkyada, and Lundberg are three manufacturers that produce rice pasta. When my first book was published the only pasta available was corn, and it was HARD to cook properly. The new rice pastas are very good. They take more time to cook but are worth it! If you go to some health food stores that focus on Gluten-free like "Whole Foods", you will find a plethora of choices.

# ✳APPENDIX B✳

**FOOD FAMILIES**
Apple —apple, crabapple, pear, quince
Arrowroot —arrowroot
Banana —banana
Berry —blackberry, boysenberry, raspberry
Blueberry (heath) - blueberry, huckleberry, cranberry
Buckwheat – buckwheat, rhubarb, garden sorrel
Caper – caper
Cashew – cashew, pistachio, mango
Chinese water chestnut – water chestnut
Citrus – grapefruit, lemon, lime, orange, tangerine
Coffee – coffee
Cola Nut (Stercula) – chocolate, cocoa, cola nut
Composite – globe artichoke, Jerusalem artichoke, chicory, endive, escarole, lettuce, safflower seed, tarragon
Crustacean – crab, lobster, shrimp
Ebony – date, plum, persimmon
Elm- slippery elm tea
Fish- all true fish; either freshwater or saltwater, including tuna, sardine, catfish, trout, and tilapia.
Fungi – mushroom, yeast
Ginger – cardamom, turmeric, ginger
Goosefoot – beet, beet sugar, spinach, Swiss chard
Gourd (melon) – cantaloupe, cucumber, honeydew, pumpkin, squash, watermelon, zucchini
Grape – raisin, grapes
Grass – wheat corn, rice, oats barley, rye, wild rice, cane sugar, millet, bamboo shoots
Honey – honey, bee nectar
Honeysuckle – elderberry
Iris – saffron
Laurel – avocado, cinnamon, bay leaves, sassafras
Legume (pea) – kidney beans, lima bean, navy bean, soy bean, carob, green pea, split pea, alfalfa, lentil, green bean
Lily – asparagus, chive, leek, onion, shallot, garlic, sarsaparilla

Linden – linden tea
Linseed – flax, flaxseed
Mallow – althea root tea, cottonseed, okra
Maple – maple sugar
Meat Family – beef (veal, dairy products, gelatin), pork, lamb
Mint – balm, basil, marjoram, rosemary, sage, thyme, savory, spearmint, mint, peppermint
Mollusk – oyster, clam, abalone, mussel
Morning Glory – sweet potato, yam
Mulberry -- breadfruit, fig, mulberry
Mustard – mustard green, cabbage, cauliflower, collard, Chinese cabbage, broccoli, brussel sprout, radish, turnip, watercress, kale
Myrtle – allspice, guava, clove
Nettle – hop, oregano
Nightshade – eggplant, cayenne, bell pepper, paprika, tomato, potato, pimento
Nutmeg – mace, nutmeg
Olive – black olive, green olive
Orchid - vanilla
Palm – coconut, dates
Parsley – anise, carrot, celery, caraway seed, parsley, coriander, dill cumin, fennel
Pepper - black and white pepper
Pineapple - pineapple
Pistachio – pistachio nuts (these are seeds from the tree)
Plum – plum, cherry, peach, apricot, nectarine, wild cherry, almond
Rose – blackthorn, strawberry
Seaweed – dulse, kelp
Sesame – sesame seed
Shellfish – oysters, scallops
 Spurge – tapioca
Tea – green tea, black tea
Walnut – English walnut, black walnut, pecan, hickory nut, butternut

# ✳APPENDIX C✳

**ALLERGY RESOURCES**

These are just a few of the many resources available

American Academy of allergy, Asthma and Immunology (AAAAI)
555 E. Wells Street
Milwaukee, WI, 53202
www.aaaai.org (800) 822-2762

American Academy of Immunologists
9650 Rockville Pike
Bethesda, MD 20892
www.aai.org (301) 634-7178

American Board of Allergy and Immunology
510 Walnut Street, Suite 1701
Philadelphia, PA 19106-3699
www.abai.org (866)264-5568

American Celiac Society Dietary Support Coalition
P.O Box 23455
New Orleans, LA 70183
amerceliac@netscape.net

American Dietetic Association
120 South Riverside Plaza, Suite 2000
Chicago, Il 60606-6995
www.eatright.org (800)877-1600

Asthma and Allergy foundation of America (AAFA)
1233 20th Street NW Suite 402
Washington, DC, 20036
www.aafa.org (202) 466-7643

The Food Allergy and Anaphylaxis Network
11781 Lee Jackson Highway, Suite 160
Fairfax, VA 22033-3309
www.foodallergy.org (703) 691-3179

Food Allergy Research and Resource program
143 H.C. Filley Hall
University of Nebraska
Lincoln, NE 68583-0919
farrp@unl.edu

Autism society of America
7910 Wood Ave., Suite 300
Bethesda, MD 20814-3015
(800) 3Autism, est. 150

Celiac Sprue Research Foundation
P.O. Box 61193
Palo Alto, CA 94306-1193
www.celiacsupport.stanford.edu

Celiac Disease Foundation
13251 Ventura Blvd, Suite 1
Studio City, Ca 91604-1638
www.celiac.org/cdf (818) 990-2354

American Diabetes, Inc
1660 Duke St.
Alexandria, VA 22314
www.diabetes.org ( 800) DIABETES

Gluten Intolerance Group of North America
1511 10th Avenue, SW., Suite A
Seattle, WA 98166
www.gluten.net (206) 246- 6652

Living Without magazine
P.O. Box 2126
Northbrook, IL 60065
www.livingwithout.com (848) 480-8810

National Foundation for Celiac Awareness
124 South Maple Street
Ambler, PA 19002
info@celiacawareness.org (215) 325-1306

North American Society for Pediatric Gastroenterology, Hepatology and Nutrition (NASPGHAN)
P.O. Box 6
Flourtown, PA 19031
www.naspghan.org (215) 233-0808

Northwest Asthma and Allergy Center
NIAID Office of Communications and Public Liaison
6610 Rockledge Drive, MSC 6612
Bethesda, MD 20892-6612
www.nwasthma.com (800) 437-4055

National Digestive Diseases Information Clearinghouse
2 Information Way
Bethesda, MD 20892-3570
nddic@info.niddk.nih.gov (800)- 891-5389

The American Gastroenterological Association
4930 Del Ray Avenue
Bethesda, MD 20814
www.gastro.org (301) – 654-2055

Intestinal Disease Foundation
Landmarks Building, Suite 525
100 West Stations Square Drive
Pittsburgh, PA 15219
www.intestinalfoundation.org

International Foundation for Functional Gastrointestinal Disorders
P.O Box 170864
Milwaukee, WI 53217
www.iffgd.org (888) 964-2001

The Joint Council of Allergy, Asthma and Immunology
50 N. Brockway, Suite 3.3
Palatine, IL 60067
info@jcaai.org (847) 934-1918

# ❋ INGREDIENT GLOSSARY ❋

## BEANS AND LEGUMES

Black beans, kidney beans, garbanzo beans (chick pea), pinto beans and lentils are all prepared by washing, shelling, and boiling for 30 minutes. But because of people's busy schedules, this is not always possible. Cans of prepared beans will be used in the recipes of this book for convenience. Refried beans may be used. This is a mixture of different beans often cooked in lard. We will be using "Vegetarian Refried beans "only.

Beans and legumes are all high in protein, yet they are still an incomplete protein. The exception to this is soybeans, the one legume that is a complete protein. Beans are a good source of soluble fiber and relatively safe for ingestion. However, some individuals are developing allergies to soy. If this allergy is suspected the recipes containing tofu and soy must be omitted.

## CHEESES

Cheese as a source of protein is too important to ignore. Therefore cheeses containing no cow's milk need to be included in the allergic individual's diet. Most individuals are not allergic but intolerant of the cow's fat molecules. The choices other than cows are: ewe (sheep), goat, reindeer and buffalo. Cheeses made from reindeer are impossible to find and we will not discuss.

True mozzarella is made from the milk of the water buffalo, a type of wild ox. Mozzarella di Buffala is different from the mozzarella found in most stores. This cheese is very white, soft but slightly firm outside. True mozzarella has hint of both sweet and sour taste. It can be found at Italian delis and is wonderful on pizzas and in salads. The whey that is left after producing mozzarella is a rare and delicious Ricotta. I have yet been able to find this Ricotta.

Goat cheeses come in many shapes and varieties. Goat's milk is not always used alone for cheeses. Sometimes it is mixed with other milks, like sheep. This should be clearly labeled. However, in the United States not all of the producers are clear what milks they are using. Beware and read the labels. The word chevre means goat and/or goat cheese. Goat cheese can be fresh or aged. It can come in different types. Newer types are Brie, Gouda, Colby, Jalapeno jack and tub cheeses flavored with herbs, hot peppers, tomatoes, fruits or honey. Goat cheese does contain lactose. But it is more easily digested than cow's milk because of the fat globules in the goat's milk do not cluster together as the cow's do.

## CHEESES MADE FOR GOAT'S MILK

**Bucheron.** A French imported cheese with a very goaty taste.

**Capricette.** Another French import, this cheese is smooth with a tangy taste.

**Chevrotins.** Also known as Chevret cheeses, the goat cheeses are popular gourmet items and expensive. The Chevrotins that are pure goat's milk are: Chevret di Comme, Chevret de Moulins, Chevret de Souvigny.

**Feta.** A cheese from Greece, which is made from ewe's milk and sometimes goat's milk. Be very careful about this cheese. I have recently seen some Feta made from cow's milk. Read the label!

**La Banion.** A French import, this cheese has a slightly nutty flavor.

**Montrachet.** This cheese is mild and creamy. It is usually served at the end of the meal. This is one of the most common goat cheeses found in the United States.

**Persilles Des Aravio.** This is a very tangy and sharp cheese. It is good as an appetizer.

**Poivre-d'Ane.** Another French import, this cheese is mild and seasoned with herbs. Beware – this cheese is sometimes mixed with cow's milk.

**Roila.** A cheese made exclusively from goat's or ewe's milk.

**Teleme.** Also known as Brandza de Braila, this cheese is produced from fresh goat's or ewe's milk.

**Valencay.** Made from raw goat's milk, this cheese has a slightly nutty taste.

**SHEEP'S MILK** (ewe) is becoming easier and more popular in the United States. The most famous of the ewe's milk cheese is Pecorino Romano, only found in Italian delis. This cheese is often used in place of Parmesan cheese.

## CHEESES MADE FROM EWE'S (SHEEP) MILK

**Annot.** This cheese is made either from sheep or goat's milk. It has a mild nutty flavor and is used in desserts.

**Feta.** A very tangy tasting cheese used in salads, breads, and entrees. In Greece this cheese is usually made from ewe's milk or goat's milk. In the United States it is made from cow's milk unless stated.

**Fontina.** This cheese, which comes from Italy, is made either from cow's or ewe's milk. In the United States it is always made from cow's milk.

**Ideazabal.** Is a smoked semisoft sheep's-milk cheese from the Basque province of Spain? It as a mild smoky and nutty flavor.

**Kasseri.** A snappy flavored cheese with a golden appearance; it is a good substitute for Parmesan cheese in recipes. This cheese, when imported from Greece, is produced from ewe's or goat's milk.

**Kafalotysi.** Another cheese from Greece, Kefalotysi is a hard cheese used mostly for grating. This cheese is produced from either ewe's or goat's milk. Surprisingly, this cheese is also produced in the Ozark region of Arkansas.

**Manchego.** This cheese comes from the center of Spain. It is zesty and can be used in place of Asiago cheese. Manchego cheese grates well. It is produced only from ewe's milk.

**Pecorino.** Also known as Pecorino Romano, Pecorino Dolco, Pecorino Grosetto, this cheese comes from Italy. All varieties are made only from ewe's milk. This cheese is normally found in Italian delis and sometimes supermarkets.

**Romano.** See Pecorino

**Roncal.** From the province of Navarre, Spain, this cheese is smooth and moist. It has a well-rounded flavor.

**Roquefort.** This cheese, which has a very pronounced taste, is used in salads, dressings, and cheese spreads. Imported from France, it is produced from raw ewe's milk.

**Serra de Estralla.** This cheese is manufactured exclusively from ewe's milk.

**Touloumiso.** This cheese is imported from Greece. The ingredients found in this cheese are identical to those found in Feta cheese.

**Zamorano.** From the province of Zamorano, Spain this sheep's cheese is semi-firm. It is similar in taste to Manchego cheese.

## EGGS

The importance of eggs as a complete protein is marred by the fact that they contain as much fat as they do protein. Most of this fat is in the yolk of the egg. Eggs are also known for their allergy potential. Generally, this is due to the protein found in the egg white. As stated in the beginning of the book. Allergy testing for egg whites should be done under a physician direction. This book only tests for the egg yolks. Until eggs are ruled out as allergy-causing, the cook should use the egg substitutes listed in Appendix A.

## FISH

Fish, especially white fish (sole, cod, snapper, tilapia, trout, turbot) is another complete protein food. Unlike meat, it contains very little fat. Fatty fish ( salmon, herring, mackerel, tuna contain a little more fat that white fish, but are still and immense improvement over red meat. Shellfish (clams, mussels, oysters, scallops) have good protein. However, crustaceans (shrimp, lobster, and crab), are known for their allergic properties. These three crustaceans will not be found in any recipes in this book.

## FLOURS

Cooking without wheat flours takes more time and attention than normal. These flours are heavier than regular flours. Therefore, you will not use as much. Tea breads and cakes do not rise as much. When cooking with these flours, you will need something to keep the breads and cakes from falling apart. That is the reason you will see xanthan gum used in every recipe.

If you want to convert a sauce recipe to wheat-free (gluten-free), it will need less white rice flour as a thickener. So start with half the recommended amount in a wheat flour recipe.

**Arrowroot.** A fine flour, used as a thickening agent, that is usually found in the spice section of the supermarket. Use like corn starch when thickening. Garbanzo bean, Potato starch, Tapioca, Sorghum or White Sorghum, and Fava Bean Flour are a group of flours used together or in other combinations for Gluten-free cooking.

**Garbanzo bean flour.** Used in combination with other flours or used for gravies in this book.

**Potato starch.** Potato starch is a very lightweight flour that is an excellent ingredient for sponge cakes, muffins, and pancakes. Most supermarkets carry it.

**Tapioca flour.** Lightweight flour, tapioca flour is made from the cassava plant. Use in combination with other flours. It is a good source of phosphorus, potassium, calcium, and magnesium. Do not use as a thickener, it is difficult to work with. It works well with baked foods.

**Sorghum or white sorghum.** Excellent flour for breading meats and used in combination with other flours for baking

**Rice Flour.** Rice flour can be white or brown flour. The white is lighter and can be used as a thickener. Use less than wheat flour. It can be used in most baking. On needs a moisture retaining flour when baking with it.

**Teff flour.** This flour has a wheat-like taste. It is high in iron content. It is related to the rice family.

**All purpose Gluten-free baking mix.** There are many types. Most use a combination of the flours listed above. Beware of Arrowhead. It contains corn starch. Use after testing for that allergen.

## GRAINS

**Buckwheat (Kasha).** Buckwheat is a grain cultivated for flour or grouts. It can be eaten as a cereal or cooked like rice. It is a good source of phosphorous and potassium. It can be found in flour form also. It is good for pancakes and waffles. Most health food stores and supermarkets carry it.

**Millet.** This grain is produced in the United States and Europe for its small edible seeds. Its protein content is higher than barley or corn. It is a good source of fiber, and is extremely rich in phosphorus, potassium, and magnesium. In flour form one can use up to 50 percent of the millet flour in exchange for wheat flour.

**Rice.** Types of rice:

**Arborio.** This is a short-grain rice of Italian origin. It is cooked slowly with heated liquid to give it a slightly soggy texture.

**Brown.** This rice is a vitamin rich food because of the bran layer has not been removed. Brown rice contains a rich supply of Vitamin B, calcium, phosphorous, and iron. It has a nice nutty flavor. Types of brown rice are: long, rose and Basmati.

**White.** White rice when processed loses 2 percent of its protein and all of its thiamine because of the hull and the bran are removed by polishing. Converted rice undergoes a similar manufacturing process, but is left with

213

higher vitamin content than white rice. Types of white rice are: Arborio, Rose, Basmati, and long Grain.

## HERBS AND SPICES

Any spice or herb might be a potential cause of an allergy. This book's recipes do contain spices and herbs. It is suggested that every spice label is read before using.

**Basil.** This herb is a member of the mint family. It has a pleasant sweet flavor. Its uses are many, especially in stews, beans, and vegetables. Soups, salads, poultry, and meats are more appealing with this seasoning.

**Bay Leaves.** This mild herb from the European Bay, Laurel or California Bay tree, is frequently used to season all types of meat, vegetables, soups, relishes, and poultry. One word of caution, Bay leaves are very sharp. Make sure you remove them before eating the meal.

**Capers.** This seasoning is a bud off a Mediterranean plant that belongs to the mustard family. Capers are often found in Italian dishes and appetizers. They are either pickled or preserved in salt.

**Fennel Seed.** This is a spice with a distinctive flavor, not unlike anise. It originated for India and parts of Bulgaria. The seeds are used in salads, vegetable dishes, and fish dished, and t spice up rolls and breads.

**Dill.** This seasoning in seed or dried weed form has a delightful flavor that tastes somewhat like parsley yet with a little more tang. Dill goes with fish, poultry, salads, and sauces. Traditionally, it is used between layers of cucumber in brine to make dill pickles.

**Italian Seasoning.** A mixture of dried herbs, containing oregano, marjoram, thyme, savory, basil, rosemary, and sage. It is usually found in the spice section of the supermarket. Check for wheat or gluten fillers in this spice.

**Marjoram.** Sweet marjoram is a subtle herb with a pleasant taste that enhances a food without altering the food's flavor. This herb is used for sauces, soups, meats, stuffing and fish.

**Mint.** An herb with the flavor of spearmint, mint does wonders for lamb dishes. It also enhances the flavor of vegetables, salads, meat broths, teas, and ices.

**Oregano.** An herb known as "joy of the mountain", oregano is indispensible in Italian, Spanish, and Greek dishes. It can be used in meat dishes, beans, soups, and sauces.

214

**Parsley.** This herb with its crisp leaves is used extensively as a garnish and seasoning. It has the added benefit of being a rich source of Vitamins C, A, and iron.

**Rosemary.** Rosemary is an evergreen often found growing along the coast of the Mediterranean. It is an herb with a powerful flavor that enriches meat dishes, sauces, greens, and stuffing.

**Sage.** Sage is a culinary herb that is satisfactory for stuffing, stews, and bean dishes. It should never be used alone, but with thyme or basil.

**Tarragon.** Tarragon is an invaluable herb for a fish sauce, for it removes the fishy odor and leaves a fresh, pleasant flavor. It is also used for poultry sauces, stews, meats, soups, and dressings. Tarragon is the most important seasoning for tartar sauce.

**Thyme.** Thyme is an evergreen with a strong, sweet flavor. It is a most versatile herb and can be found in soups, sauces, stuffing, spreads, meats, fish, poultry, and dressings. It is usually used in tomato dishes or dishes with tomato sauce.

## LIQUIDS

**Almond Breeze.** An Almond drink made from almonds and purified water. It contains soy.

**Rice Dream.** This drink is made from filtered water and brown rice.

**Soy milk.** Soy milk is made from organic soybeans and filtered water. Soy milk is low in fat and carbohydrates. It is rich in thiamine, niacin, and calcium.

**Non-citrus Juices.** Example of such juices are "pure" apple juice, pear, apricot, and cranberry juice.

## MEATS

**Lamb and Beef.** Both lamb and beef contain protein, B vitamins, and iron. Like dairy products, meats are complete protein foods. Unfortunately, they are also high in saturated fats. When selecting a meat (lamb or beef), choose lean meat. When selecting cured meat, choose a kosher brand. Kosher meats do not have any milk or milk by-products in the meat. When preparing the meat, be sure that all meats are cooked to at least a pink color. Rare meats tend to cause headaches.

## MUSHROOMS

A mushroom is a type of fungus generally found in cool damp places where the soil is rich. A mushroom consists of a stalk and umbrella-shaped cap. Although many mushrooms have high water content, they have a greater food value than green vegetables. The parasol mushrooms are protein-rich and are considered gastronomic prizes as food. Some of the gourmet types of mushrooms are: Portabella, Crimini, Enoki, Porcini, Shiitake, Wood ear, Morel, and Chanterelles.

**Chanterelle:** This mushroom is trumpet-shaped and has a chewy texture and delicate flavor. Its color ranges from golden to yellow orange.

**Crimini:** The crimini mushroom is a brown variety of the button mushroom.

**Enoki:** This mushroom has a tiny cap and grows in clumps. It has very long, slender stems. This mushroom is very flavorful for salads.

**Morel:** This mushroom has an elongated honeycomb shape. It has a rich, smoky flavor. It can be found fresh or dried.

**Oyster:** This is an oriental mushroom. It has a short stem and ragged edged shape resembling an oyster

**Porcini:** This mushroom can be found fresh or dried. It has a wonderful rich nutty flavor. This brown mushroom is also called cepe.

**Portobello:** Sometimes spelled portabella, this mushroom is very popular for its meaty taste. The mushroom has a large cap with exposed gills that are sometimes removed before cooking.

**Shiitake:** This popular oriental mushroom has a cap that is floppy and flat. It has a rich meaty flavor. It can be found fresh or dried.

**Wood Ear:** This is another oriental mushroom with a wonderful flavor. It resembles large, floppy brown ears. Dried it looks like wood chips. This mushroom is also known as cloud ear or tree ear.

## NUTS

**Almonds.** Although the almond really belongs to the plum family, it is still classified as a nut. Almonds are rich in protein and unsaturated fats. Almonds contain high amounts of phosphorus, potassium, and calcium. When almonds are referred to in the recipe section, the almonds should be roasted or toasted to remove any oils or extracts.

**Pine Nuts.** Pine Nuts (or pignoles) are another mislabeled nut. Pine nuts are really seeds of the Stone Pine tree. Rich in iron, potassium, and phosphorous, these "nuts" are 31 percent protein. Pine Nuts are used in Italian, **Greek and middle Eastern cooking.** These seeds are about ½ inch ling with a delicate flavor that enhances most entrees.

**Pistachio.** Pistachio nuts are really seeds from the Pistachio tree. This tree, native to the Near East, is now cultivated in the Mediterranean and southern United States. The nut is enclosed in a brownish shell that is easy to open. Pistachio nuts are rich in fat and carbohydrates. The nuts are used for decorating foods and for sauces and soups.

## OILS AND MARGARINES

**Olive oil.** This monounsaturated oil contains only 10 percent of the necessary fatty acid, linoleic acid. It also has more calories than butter or lard. This oil is usually found in Italian, Greek and other Mediterranean dishes.

**Safflower oil (or margarine).** This cold pressed, polyunsaturated natural oil contains 70-50 percent of the fatty acid, linoleic acid. Safflower oil is a good source of Vitamin E.

**Soybean oil (or margarine).** This is polyunsaturated oil is used sparingly with other oils. It is found mostly in Oriental and Indonesian dishes.

## POULTRY

**Turkey and Chicken.** Poultry is another complete protein food. It is low in saturated fats. This book requests that male birds be used in most recipe dishes. Try to buy Organic Chicken that has not been given hormones.

## SOYBEAN PRODUCTS AND SEASONINGS

**Miso.** Known also as bean curd paste, miso is a high-protein seasoning produced by soybeans. Like yogurt, it contains lactobacillus and other healthful bacteria regarded as beneficial to the intestine. The Japanese use it as a basic staple as it is a concentrated source of protein. Miso is used along with tamari-like bouillon in soups and stews, and like Worcestershire in sauces, dressings and dips. Brown rice miso is the miso of choice. It has a deep, rich flavor and a pleasant fragrance. This particular type of miso contains 12 -14 percent protein and is relatively easy to find.

**Tamari.** Tamari is a seasoning that is much richer than most soy sauces. Use it sparingly. The organic variety normally does not contain wheat. Check that labels.

**Tofu.** Also known as soybean curd, this is made from the only legume that is a complete protein. It is a common food of the traditional Oriental diet and often referred to as "the meat without a Bone". More varieties of tofu are available for cooking. Some forms such as tofutti can be used instead of cream cheese or sour cream.

## SWEETENERS

**Honey.** Honey is almost twice as sweet as cane or beet sugar. Smaller amounts are needed for sweetening. However, the sources and production of honey is such a variable that it limits its uses in hypoallergenic cooking.

**Molasses (blackstrap).** This is the last substance left after the extraction of sugar form the sugar cane. It is a rich source of vitamins and minerals especially iron.

**Maple syrup.** This is usually a solution of dissolved sugar with maple extract. Maple syrup in its pure form can be found in health food stores.

**Rice syrup.** This is a new form of sweetening that can be substituted for honey, corn syrup, sugar and molasses. The amount used is more rice syrup and less sugar or other sweetener. It has not been used too much as of yet. But I think it will make a big difference in allergy food sweetening.

**Sugar.** Sugar is a sweet, crystalline substance obtained from the juice of the sugar cane or sugar beet. It is a major carbohydrate source lacking any protein, vitamins, or minerals.

# ❋BIBLIOGRAPHY❋

## BOOKS

Androque, Pierre. The complete Encyclopedia of French cheese. New York: Harper's Magazine Press, 1973

Balch, Phyllis A., Balch, James, F MD. Prescription for Nutritional Healing. New York; Avery, 2000

Editors of Cook's Illustrated. The New Best Recipe. Massachusetts; American Test Kitchens, 2007

Fenster, Carol, PHD. Wheat-free Recipes and Menus. New York; Avery, 2004

Lang, Jennifer H. Larousse Gastronomique. New York; Crown Publishers, Inc., 1999

Lowell, Jax P. the gluten-free bible. New York; Henry Wolf and Company, 2005

Giann, Allen V. The Best Guide to Allergy. New York; Appleton-Century Crofts, 1981

Kirschman, Gayla J., Kirschman, James D. Nutritional Almanac. New York; McGraw-Hill, 1996

Null, Gary. Get Healthy Now. New York; Seven Stories Press, 1999

Salt II MD, William B. IBS and the Mind-Body Brain-Gut Connection. Ohio; Parkview Publishing, 1997

Van Vorous, Heather. Eating for IBS. New York; Marlow and Company, 2000

editors of, The Cheese Bible. New York; Penguin Studio, 1998

Walsh MD, William E. Food Allergies: The Complete Guide to Understanding and Relieving Your Food Allergies. New York; John Wiley and Sons, Inc, 2000

## ARTICLES

Altman Dr, Chiaramonte LT. Public perception of food allergy. J Allergy Clin Immunol. Jun 1996;97

Bai JC, Vazquez H, Nachman F, et al. Novel antibody tests based on synthetic gliadin-related peptides have a great yield for celiac disease. Gastroenterology. 2006;133 (Abstract)

Bock SA, Atkins FM. Patterns of food hypersensitivity during sixteen years of double-blind, placebo-controlled food challenges. J Pediatrics. Oct. 1990;117

James JM, Burks AW. Food-associated gastrointestinal disease. Curr Opin Pediatr. Oct 1996; 8

Lever R, MacDonald C, Waugh P, AitchisonT. Randomized controlled trial of advice on egg exclusion diet in young children with atopic eczema and sensitivity to eggs. Pediatr Allergy Immunol. Feb 1998;9

Lohi S, Mustalahti K, Kaukinen K, et al. The prevalence of celiac disease is increasing in process of time. Gastroenterology. 2006; 130 (Abstract)

Roberts G, Patel N, Levi-Schaffer F et al. Food allergy as a risk factor for life-threatening asthma in childhood: a case-controlled study. J Allergy Clin Immunol. Jul 2003;112

**INTERNET SOURCES**

1. www.arby's.com
2. www.bajafresh.com
3. www.burgerking.com
4. www.carl'sjr.com
5. www.chipotle.com
6. www.deltaco.com
7. www.elpolloloco.com
8. www.inandoutburger.com
9. www.jackinthebox.com
10. www.mcdonald's.com
11. www.pandaexpress.com
12. www.sonicdrivein.com
13. www.tacobell.com
14. www.wendy's.com
15. www.glutenfreeceliacweb.com
16. www.celiaccentral.org
17. www.glutenfreeonthego.com
18. www.celiacofeasternpa.com
19. www.gluten.nd/safe-dining.htm